Treating Adolescents
with Substance Use Disorders

Treating Adolescents with Substance Use Disorders

Oscar G. Bukstein

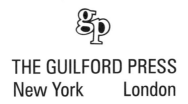

THE GUILFORD PRESS
New York   London

Printed in the United States of America

This book is printed on acid-free paper.

Last digit is print number: 9 8 7 6 5 4 3 2 1

The author has checked with sources believed to be reliable in his efforts to provide
information that is complete and generally in accord with the standards of practice that
are accepted at the time of publication. However, in view of the possibility of human error
or changes in behavioral, mental health, or medical sciences, neither the author, nor
the editor and publisher, nor any other party who has been involved in the preparation
or publication of this work warrants that the information contained herein is in every
respect accurate or complete, and they are not responsible for any errors or omissions
or the results obtained from the use of such information. Readers are encouraged to
confirm the information contained in this book with other sources.

Library of Congress Cataloging-in-Publication Data

Names: Bukstein, Oscar Gary, 1955– author.
Title: Treating adolescents with substance use disorders / Oscar G. Bukstein.
Description: New York : The Guilford Press, [2019] | Includes bibliographical references
   and index.
Identifiers: LCCN 2019013022 | ISBN 9781462537860 (hardback)
Subjects: LCSH: Teenagers—Substance use—Treatment. | Substance abuse. |
   BISAC: PSYCHOLOGY / Psychopathology / Addiction. | MEDICAL / Psychiatry /
   Child & Adolescent. | SOCIAL SCIENCE / Social Work. | PSYCHOLOGY /
   Psychotherapy / Child & Adolescent.
Classification: LCC RJ506.D78 B853 2019 | DDC 616.8600835—dc23
LC record available at *https://lccn.loc.gov/2019013022*

About the Author

Oscar G. Bukstein, MD, MPH, is Vice-Chair of Psychiatry at Boston Children's Hospital and Professor of Psychiatry at Harvard Medical School. Previously, he was Professor of Psychiatry and Chief of the Division of Child and Adolescent Psychiatry at the University of Texas Health Science Center at Houston and Medical Director of DePelchin Children's Center. Dr. Bukstein spent 28 years at the Western Psychiatric Institute and Clinic and the University of Pittsburgh School of Medicine, where he achieved the rank of Professor of Psychiatry. Since the 1980s, his clinical practice and research have focused on treatment of youth with substance use disorders and other disruptive behavior disorders. He has authored or coauthored over 150 papers, chapters, or books. Dr. Bukstein is co-chair of the Committee on Quality Issues of the American Academy of Child and Adolescent Psychiatry, which develops clinical practice guidelines for professionals treating children and adolescents with psychiatric disorders.

Preface

Having published widely on substance use disorders (SUDs) in adolescents, I knew my next book would focus on helping therapists to work effectively with these hard-to-treat teens. My previous books may have furthered our understanding of critical research in the field, but they did not answer the question posed by many of my trainees: "What do I do now?" What my previous books, chapters, and papers did not offer was the means to assimilate the information into a useful, practical guide to intervening in clinical contexts for problem behaviors in adolescents. I hope that this book will help therapists know what to do when they are faced with a client in their offices, clinics, and inpatient units.

WHAT THIS BOOK OFFERS

While many of the strategies in this book have been influenced by treatment manuals for evidence-based interventions, I have distilled the research literature and these manuals to provide readers with a general clinical approach for working with adolescents and their families in evaluation and treatment of SUDs.

More specifically, there are common characteristics across effective therapies, including the importance of motivation and engagement, developing a variety of recovery skills, paying attention to family issues (particularly parent management of adolescents and improving parent–adolescent communication and problem solving), developing a prosocial peer network, and considering coexisting mental health problems. This book covers each of these areas, along with a variety of techniques. Each chapter tries to provide the reader with answers to the question "Given what the literature currently says, what should the clinician do in assessing and treating adolescents with SUDs?"

Chapter 1 provides background about adolescents with SUDs, including important risk factors and the evidence base for interventions. Chapter 2 describes approaches and strategies for motivating and engaging teens and their parents. Chapters 3 and 4 discuss the process and content, respectively, of screening and assessment, where motivational strategies are key from the first encounter. Chapter 5 covers treatment planning and brief interventions. It includes an outline for a brief, four-session treatment course appropriate for adolescents with mild to moderate substance use problems. Chapter 6 describes a group intervention for teaching adolescents recovery skills such as functional analysis, problem solving, coping with urges, relapse prevention, and increasing prosocial behaviors and peer relationships. Chapter 7 focuses on a six-session parent management training group that teaches how to monitor teens, use contingency management and positive reinforcement, and develop communication skills. Chapter 8 describes the family intervention called parent–adolescent problem solving. Teens who have learned recovery and communication skills and parents who have undergone parent management training are usually ready to meet together in joint sessions to solve problems and negotiate contracts. Chapter 9 addresses the issue of how treatment for SUDs can be integrated with treatments for comorbid psychiatric disorders. Finally, a brief epilogue ends the volume with a look at prevention of SUDs.

A few comments about the language and labels used in this book are in order. While I make use of a variety of terms to describe substance use, I have adopted the current diagnostic label of "substance use disorders," abbreviated "SUDs," from the fifth edition of the *Diagnostic and Statistical Manual of Mental Disorders* (DSM-5; American Psychiatric Association, 2013), to refer to the pathological pattern of substance use. I have attempted to minimize my use of such general terms as "addiction" or "substance abuse." I have also attempted to keep citations to the literature to a minimum, summarizing research where possible, but also providing references when citing a specific finding. For those readers desiring more information, the Appendix includes books, papers, organizations, and relevant websites that provide a wide variety of information about the science and clinical care of adolescents with SUDs.

All of the clinical examples in the book are fictionalized and are not based on any real persons.

Acknowledgments

In the course of my career, I have been very fortunate to benefit from the wisdom and assistance of many of my colleagues. At the University of Pittsburgh, I first want to thank David Brent, an inspiration, primary mentor, and friend; and Brooke Molina, a valued colleague and friend whose help has figured greatly in the content of this volume. Others include Duncan Clark, Tammy Chung, Jack Cornelius, Dennis Daley, Thomas Kelly, David Kolko, the late Rolf Loeber, Boris Birmaher, David Axelson, Ralph Tarter, Sharon Levy, and my old boss David Kupfer. A number of other colleagues also deserve thanks, including William Pelham, Benjamin Goldstein, Deborah Deas, Paula Riggs, Yifrah Kaminer, and Vincent Van Hasselt.

A special thanks to my former coordinators, Heidi Kipp and Jennifer Baker, without whose help . . . well, I would have gotten very little done. Of course, I appreciate the efforts of the folks at The Guilford Press, particularly Kitty Moore, Senior Editor, who exhibited great patience and provided much encouragement.

Finally, I am grateful to my wife, Adrienne, for her support and patience.

Contents

1. Adolescents with Substance Use Disorders: 1
How Did They Get There?
The Specific Treatments That Work for Adolescents with SUDs 9
Pharmacological Treatments for SUDs 13
From Evidence-Based Interventions to Practice 15

2. Motivation and Engagement 17
Parent and Family Motivation and Engagement 18
Motivational Interviewing 23
Contingency Management 41
Summary 43

3. The Process of Screening and Assessment 44
Gateways to Screening and Assessment 45
Confidentiality 53
The Role of Parents in the Assessment Process 54
Engaging the Parents 55
Interviewing and Engaging Adolescents 56
Drug Testing 62
Summary 64

4. The Content of Screening and Assessment　　　65

Screening　65
The Comprehensive Assessment　78
Summary　91

5. Treatment Planning and Brief Interventions　　　92

Who Can Treat Adolescents with SUDs?　92
Elements of Effective Treatment　93
Responding to Parent Concerns　97
Levels of Care　98
Brief Interventions　101
Outpatient Treatment　106
Intensive Outpatient Treatment　107
Residential Levels of Care　107
Aftercare　108
Alternative Peer-Group Programs　110
Recovery High Schools　111
Adequate Duration of Treatment　111
Twelve-Step Interventions　112
Group Treatment　115
Cultural Factors　117

6. Cognitive-Behavioral Recovery Skills　　　121

Key Components of CBT for Adolescents with SUDs　122
CBT for Adolescents with SUDs　130
Summary　163

7. Parent Management Training　　　164

Elements of a Family-Based Behavioral Therapy　165
PMT for Parents of Adolescents with SUDs　168
Summary　188

8. Parent–Adolescent Problem Solving　　　189

Parent–Adolescent Negotiation　190
Modification of Parent–Adolescent Negotiation　207
Summary　208

9. Integrated Treatment for Substance Use Disorders
and Other Psychiatric Disorders 209

Can Substance Use and Psychiatric Treatments Coexist? *210*
Approaches to the Treatment of Comorbid Disorders
in Adolescents *212*
Summary and Recommendations *230*

Epilogue 231

Prevention *232*
Conclusion *232*

Appendix. Resources 237

Internet Resources *237*
Treatment Manuals *239*

References 241

Index 260

Purchasers can download and print enlarged versions
of the reproducible figures at *www.guilford.com/bukstein-forms* for
personal use or use with clients (see copyright page for details).

Chapter One

Adolescents with Substance Use Disorders
How Did They Get There?

A ccumulating evidence regarding physical maturation suggests that adolescence is distinctly different from adulthood. Specific areas of the brain have yet to fully complete their development, which has a host of clinical implications. The past 150 years have also witnessed a quiet but dramatic change in human development: children are growing faster, reaching reproductive and physical maturity at earlier ages, and often growing to be taller than perhaps at any time in human history. Adolescence has expanded from perhaps a 2- to 4-year interval in traditional societies to as much as an 8-year interval. Most importantly, the adolescent brain does not reach full maturity and metacognition—the ability to think about one's actions in a more considered way—until age 25. All of these new changes affect adolescents' decisions about alcohol and drug use.

This chapter presents an overview of adolescent substance use and misuse. Prevalence of their use as well as gender differences are presented, along with neurocognitive and developmental considerations. This chapter also provides an overview of available interventions, spanning individual, family, and pharmacological treatment options, and describes the scientific evidence regarding the efficacy of these approaches. The purpose is to gain a general understanding of the evidence base of the development and treatment of substance use disorders (SUDs) with the ultimate goal of the clinician's increased appreciation of why we should approach the treatment of adolescents in the manner that we propose in this book. Providing a detailed discussion of the research literature

1

on epidemiology, etiology, and treatment of adolescent SUDs is beyond the scope of this book. Readers are directed to other sources, such as the references in this chapter, for additional discussions about the etiology and prevalence of these pervasive problems. In addition, readers who are familiar with this information can skip ahead to Chapter 2, in which I begin the discussion of clinical management of adolescents with SUDs.

1. **Many adolescents use one or more substances of abuse such as alcohol, marijuana, and opioids. Fewer, but overall a substantial number, meet criteria for an SUD.** Despite the fact that we will not provide an extensive overview, knowledge of the overall prevalence and patterns of use across time is potentially useful to those dealing with adolescents. These statistics are based on the most widely respected survey of drug and alcohol use among adolescents, the Monitoring the Future Survey (MFS), which has annually surveyed 8th, 10th, and 12th graders since 1975 (Johnston et al., 2018).

- Almost a quarter of today's 8th graders have tried an illicit drug (including inhalants), and nearly half of 12th graders have done so.
- One in every 17 12th graders currently smokes marijuana daily.
- The proportion of young people using *any illicit drug* (including marijuana) rose gradually from 2008 to 2011, owing largely to increased use of marijuana—the most widely used of all the illicit drugs—but remained stable to 2017. In 2017, 50% of high school seniors reported having tried an illicit drug at some time, 41.2% used one or more drugs in the past 12 months, and 25.7% used one or more drugs in the prior 30 days.
- 16.6% of 12th graders consumed five or more drinks in a row at least once in the 2 weeks prior to the survey.
- Smoking rates among American adolescents have declined over more than a decade. In the National Youth Tobacco Survey (NYTS), the percentage of students reporting current use of cigarettes declined from 15.8% in 2011 to 9.2% in 2014 (Arrazola et al., 2015).
- The NYTS revealed that e-cigarette use among youth in middle and high school almost tripled, from 4.5% in 2013 to 13.4% in 2014 (Arrazola et al., 2015). The dual use of e-cigarettes and conventional cigarettes is high among adolescents and is increasing.

For more than a decade—from the late 1970s to the early 1990s—the use of a number of illicit drugs declined appreciably among 12th-grade students in the MFS and declined even more among American college students and young adults. These substantial improvements, which were largely due to changes in attitudes about drug use, beliefs about the risks of drug use, and peer norms against drug use, have some extremely important clinical and policy implications. For the clinician, changing beliefs of the adolescent about the negative effects of substances on the adolescent and his or her peer group is an important task.

Despite the substantial improvement in the drug situation in the United States in the 1980s and early 1990s, and some further improvement beginning in the late 1990s, U.S. secondary school students and young adults continue to show a level of involvement with illicit drugs that is among the highest in the world's industrialized nations (Johnston, O'Malley, Bachman, & Schulenberg, 2011). Although in general the rates of usage of illicit drugs are not as high as in the peak years of the epidemic in the late 1970s, even by longer-term historical standards in the United States, these rates remain extremely high.

As of September 1, 2018, recreational marijuana is legal in nine states and medical marijuana is legal in 30 states in the United States, and as of October 2018, marijuana is legal in Canada. Early findings indicate that adolescent marijuana use has increased in some states postlegalization (Hall & Weier, 2017). Long-term consequences of legalization such as possible increases in the rates of cannabis use disorder in adolescents await further research regarding consequences as additional states legalize marijuana. Legalization does portend more availability of marijuana to adolescents.

As clinicians, we are mainly concerned with those adolescents who have problems with substance use. The prevalence of SUDs increases with age through young adulthood. The National Survey on Drug Use and Health (NSDUH; Substance Abuse and Mental Health Services Administration [SAMHSA], 2017) showed that the rate of illicit drug dependence or abuse among youth ages 12–17 was 3.2% in 2012. The rate of alcohol dependence or abuse among youth ages 12–17 was 2.0 %. Results from the National Comorbidity Survey—Adolescent Supplement found an overall lifetime SUD prevalence of 8.9–11.4% of adolescents with drug abuse/dependence and 6.4% with alcohol abuse/dependence (Swendsen et al., 2012). The prevalence of DSM-IV-TR-defined SUDs for illicit drugs was 3.4% in youth ages 13–14 years and 16.5% in the 17- to 18-year age group. The median age of onset for illicit drug use was 13 years, the median age for drug abuse with dependence was 14 years, and the median age for drug abuse without dependence was 15 years. In the National Comorbidity Survey, for SUDs, 5.2% of all adolescents met the criteria for alcohol abuse without dependence and 1.3% met the criteria for abuse with dependence. The rate for abuse with or without dependence was 1.3% for adolescents ages 13–14 and 15.1% for adolescents ages 17–18. Changes in diagnosis according to DSM-5 criteria are discussed in Chapter 3.

Recent national survey data indicate little to no difference in rates of past-year SUD prevalence by gender for alcohol or illicit drugs. Similar to ethnic differences in substance use prevalence among adults, larger proportions of Caucasian and Hispanic youth ages 12–17 years met the criteria for a past-year DSM-IV (no data are available for DSM-5) alcohol or drug diagnosis than African Americans (10%, 10%, and 6%, respectively), although Native American adolescents had the highest proportion of alcohol or other drug diagnoses (20%).

2. **While aspects of brain development may place adolescents in general at risk for substance use and the development of SUDs, specific risk or protective factors may place certain adolescents at higher or lower risk, respectively, for the development of SUDs.** Because of relatively immature brain development and less cognitive control, along with high urges and capacity for risk-taking behavior, adolescents may be more susceptible to a more rapid development of SUDs and consequences from substance use. Problems that further diminish cognitive controls, such as attention-deficit/hyperactivity disorder (ADHD), place the adolescent at even greater risk for the early onset of SUDs.

Despite evidence for such problems as increased conflicts with parents, mood lability and volatility, and increased risk behaviors and sensation seeking, most adolescents navigate through this period with minimal problems. Many *do* struggle with their developmental tasks. Overall, morbidity and mortality rates increase 200–300% between middle childhood and late adolescence/early adulthood. Many adolescents will exhibit the onset of problems such as cigarette and other tobacco use and nicotine dependence, alcohol and drug use, and poor health habits that will show up as mortality in adulthood. Many adult-onset psychiatric disorders such as depression can be traced to early episodes in adolescence.

But which adolescents make the occasional poor decision, and which make more pervasive ones with significant consequences? Researchers have identified the specific characteristics of an adolescent, his or her family, peers, or environment that increase the likelihood that he or she will develop problems like substance use and SUDs. These characteristics are *risk factors*. Those characteristics that make such poor outcomes less likely are termed *protective factors*. Clinicians need to be aware of risk factors, as they are often the basic targets for treatment. Similarly, clinicians can foster protective factors in adolescents to build resilience and develop skills, characteristics, knowledge, and relationships that offset risk factors. Risk factors are seen in several life domains relevant to the adolescent, including individual, family, peer, and community domains.

Protective factors are adolescent characteristics associated with a reduced likelihood of SUDs or that reduce a risk factor's impact (SAMHSA, 2017). Examples of *individual-level protective factors* include positive self-image, self-control, or social competence. *Community-level protective factors* include the availability of faith-based resources and after-school activities. *Familial protective factors* include parental involvement and the use of monitoring and other positive disciplinary practices. Protective factors are often positively correlated with one another and negatively correlated to risk factors. Adolescents with some risk factors have a greater chance of experiencing even more risk factors, and they are less likely to have protective factors. Risk and protective factors also tend to have a cumulative effect on the development—or reduced development—of behavioral health issues. Just as adolescents with multiple risk factors have a greater likelihood of developing SUDs, youth with multiple protective factors are at a reduced risk. Both prevention and treatment interventions are seen as not only targeting risk factors but also promoting protective factors.

Within a developmental context, an individual adolescent's genetic predisposition to substance use, as evidenced by the risk factors of parental SUDs, is exacerbated by environmental and individual characteristics, family issues, and peer factors (see Table 1.1). Both temperament and social interactions (i.e., family, peer relations) play a critical role in adolescent SUD outcomes. First, experiences with substance use most often take place in a social context. Adolescents at high risk for development of SUDs show an earlier attachment to peers and a decreased attachment to family relative to normal developmental trends. Having weak ties to positive influences outside the family is associated with deviant outcomes in adolescence. For example, lack of commitment to school and poor school achievement have been consistently linked to truancy, drug use, and general delinquency (Steinberg, Fletcher, & Darling, 1994). Association with antisocial peers is one of the most powerful precursors of drug use and other behavioral problems (Doran, Luczak, Bekman, Koutsenek, & Brown, 2012).

Moreover, the earlier the age of access to and onset of substance use, the more salient both environmental and constitutional risk factors become. The early onset of substance use and a more rapid progression through the stages of substance use are among the risk factors for development of SUDs (Grant & Dawson, 1998). Initiation and early patterns of use are strongly influenced by social, familial, and environmental factors, while later levels of use are strongly influenced by genetic factors (Kendler, Schmitt, Aggen, & Prescott, 2008).

Numerous factors can modify both the effect of the substance and the adolescent's experience of the substance use. Compared with adults, adolescents often experience difficulty gauging the relative risks associated with myriad behaviors, including amounts and types of substance use. Adolescents may be much less aware of signs of their own intoxication or impairment. The adolescent user may experience an extreme level of distress, particularly agitation and anxiety. These reactive, dysphoric

TABLE 1.1. Risk Factors for SUDs

Family risk factors

- Parental drug and alcohol use.
- Parental favorable attitudes toward alcohol and/or drug use.
- Marital conflict.
- Negative events.
- Family dysfunction, disturbed family environment.
- Poor parenting, rejection, lack of parental warmth.
- Permissive parenting.
- Lack of or inconsistent discipline.
- Parent–child conflict.
- Parental hostility/low attachment.
- Harsh discipline.
- Child abuse or maltreatment.
- Substance use among siblings.
- Inadequate supervision and monitoring.
- Low parental aspirations for child.

Individual risk factors

- Difficult temperament/inflexibility, low positive mood, withdrawal.
- Irritability.
- Motor, language, and cognitive impairments.
- Early aggressive behavior.
- Poor social skills: impulsive, aggressive, passive, and withdrawn.
- Poor social problem-solving skills.
- Poor impulse control/impulsivity.
- Sensation seeking.
- Lack of behavioral self-control.
- Early persistent behavior problems/antisocial behavior.
- ADHD.
- Poor concentration.
- Low self-esteem, perceived incompetence, negative explanatory and inferential style.
- Poor grades/achievements/school failure.
- Low commitment to school.

Peer risk factors

- Deviant peer group.
- Peer attitudes toward drugs.
- Decrease in social support accompanying entry into a new social context.
- Negative life events.
- Attending college.
- Substance-using peers.
- Social adversity.

(continued)

TABLE 1.1. *(continued)*

Community risk factors

- Laws and norms favorable to alcohol and drug use.
- Availability of and access to alcohol.
- Urban setting.
- Poverty.
- Community violence.
- School violence.

Protective factors

- Academic success and investment in school.
- Involvement in recreational activities.
- Association with prosocial peers.
- Stable, secure attachment to parent/caretaker.
- Consistent discipline and monitoring of activities.
- Good self-regulation, coping, and problem-solving skills.

Note. Data from National Research Council and Institute of Medicine (2009) and O'Connell, Boat, and Warner (2009).

states compound the direct neuropharmacological effects of a substance use episode.

The capacity of a specific substance to induce a pattern of repeated use in an adolescent is determined by the reinforcing effects of that substance on the particular adolescent. Reinforcing effects differ among adolescents and likely differ between adolescents and adults. Sometimes the reward is a pleasurable feeling or sometimes relief from an aversive mood state (i.e., negative reinforcement). Expectations regarding use and the social context in which adolescents use drugs and alcohol can also mediate pharmacological interactions (Smith, Goldman, Greenbaum, & Christiansen, 1995), which can result in emotional, cognitive, and behavioral changes. Adolescents' expectations of the effects of substance consumption are often different from those of adults, which will affect the adolescents' decision to use. Given their lack of knowledge and experience, their expectations can be incorrect and promote problem use. Young people may emphasize beliefs that alcohol is an aphrodisiac, an analgesic, or a social lubricant but may minimize factors such as disinhibition and/or aggressive behavior. Having an adolescent realistically consider these expectations is a part of cognitive-behavioral therapy (CBT; see Chapter 6).

3. **Clinicians should use evidence-based treatments and practices as a basis for interventions for adolescents with SUDs.** Reviews of studies of adolescent treatment outcome have concluded that treatment for adolescent SUDs is better than no treatment (Williams & Chang, 2000;

Tanner-Smith, Wilson, & Lipsey, 2013). In the year following treatment, adolescents report decreased heavy drinking, decreased marijuana and other illicit drug use, and decreased criminal involvement, as well as improved psychological adjustment and school performance (Grella, Hser, Joshi, & Rounds-Bryant, 2001; Hser et al., 2001). Longer duration of treatment is associated with more favorable outcomes (Hser et al., 2001; Tanner-Smith et al., 2013). Although the majority of treated adolescents return to some substance use following treatment, treated adolescents generally show reductions in substance use and problems over both short- and longer-term follow-up (e.g., Chung et al., 2003; Williams & Chang, 2000). Some reviews have identified such variables as co-occurring psychopathology, nonwhite race, higher severity of substance use, criminality, and lower educational status as predicting poorer adolescent SUD outcomes. The provision of comprehensive services such as housing, academic assistance, posttreatment association with nonusing peers, and involvement in leisure-time activities, work, and school predicted more positive outcomes (American Academy of Child and Adolescent Psychiatry, 2005). Other past studies reported treatment completion, low pretreatment use, peer and parent social support, and nonuse of substances to be most consistently related to positive outcomes for adolescents receiving SUD treatment (Grella et al., 2001). A more recent meta-analysis did not find any of these variables predicting improved treatment outcomes (Tanner-Smith et al., 2013).

Improvements following SUD treatment extend beyond changes in substance use. Following treatment, teens with low substance involvement generally had better psychosocial functioning at young adult follow-up compared to teens with moderate to high levels of posttreatment substance involvement (e.g., Brown, D'Amico, McCarthy, & Tapert, 2001). Worse outcomes among heavier users may reflect the impact of greater baseline impairment and the presence of co-occurring psychopathology (e.g., conduct problems). Changes in different domains of psychosocial functioning often occur at different rates. For example, in several studies, school functioning improved within the first year of follow-up, but improvements in family functioning emerged only after 2 years (Chung et al., 2003). Despite significant reductions in substance involvement and improvements in areas of school performance, other areas of functioning, such as interpersonal relations, continued to show greater problem severity across multiple domains compared to a community control group (Chung & Martin, 2005). Thus, adolescent-onset SUD, likely in combination with co-occurring psychopathology and other risk factors (e.g., negative environmental influences), appears to interfere with the achievement of some normative developmental tasks during adolescence, despite post-SUD treatment success.

Pretreatment, during-treatment, and posttreatment variables have been examined as predictors of clinical course. The most robust pretreatment characteristics predicting more persistent levels of substance involvement typically included the presence of co-occurring psychopathology (e.g., Grella et al., 2001; Tomlinson, Brown, & Abrantes, 2004). Treatment factors associated with better outcomes included greater readiness to change, that is, higher motivation (e.g., Chung, Maisto, Cornelius, & Martin, 2004). In addition, longer duration of treatment (e.g., Hser et al., 2001) and family involvement in treatment (Liddle & Dakof, 1995) predicted better outcomes. Posttreatment factors associated with better outcomes, including aftercare involvement (e.g., Winters, Stinchfield, & Opland, 2000), low levels of peer substance use (e.g., Winters et al., 2000), and continued commitment to abstain (Kelly, Myers, & Brown, 2000), accounted for more of the variance in outcome over 1-year follow-up than pre- and during-treatment factors (Hsieh, Hoffmann, & Hollister, 1998).

THE SPECIFIC TREATMENTS THAT WORK FOR ADOLESCENTS WITH SUDs

The findings noted above relate to the treatment of adolescents with SUDs in general. In a variety of clinical trials, investigators have studied specific modalities and models of treatment.

Treatment effects can be moderated by age, ethnicity, comorbidity, level of impairment, and affiliation with delinquent peers. Among the most important pretreatment moderators of treatment is the presence of disruptive behavior problems, which appear better addressed with family-based interventions than individual or group-based models (Hendriks, van der Schee, & Blanken, 2012; Ryan, Stranger, Thostenson, Whitmore, & Budney, 2013). Similarly, adolescents with greater clinical severity or complexity, such as psychiatric comorbidity, may require more comprehensive interventions such as integrated models mentioned above. Evidence-based therapies are listed in Table 1.2.

Brief Treatments

While a robust research literature supports the effectiveness of brief interventions for alcohol use among U.S. college students and provides some models for younger teens, the college experience represents a unique social environment that might not generalize to the adolescent context. Brief interventions (BIs) with adolescents are typically between one and four sessions and can be stand-alone or part of ongoing care, usually as lead-in interventions. For example, common applications of BIs for adolescents

TABLE 1.2. Evidence-Based Treatment for Adolescents with SUDs

Intervention	Type	Population	Reference
Adolescent community reinforcement approach (A-CRA)	Family	Youth ages 13–17; girls/ boys; outpatient/home	Godley et al. (2007)
Assertive adolescent outpatient (OP) and intensive outpatient (IOP) treatment model	Individual/ group	Youth ages 12–18	Godley et al. (2010)
Brief strategic family therapy (BSFT)	Family	Youth ages 13–17; girls/ boys; outpatient/home	Santisteban et al. (1996)
Family behavior therapy (FBT)	Family	Youth ages 13–17; girls/ boys; outpatient/home	Donohue & Azrin (2011)
Family support network	Family	Youth ages 13–17; girls/ boys; outpatient/home	Dennis et al. (2004)
Functional family therapy (FFT)	Family	Youth ages 13–17; girls/ boys; outpatient/home	Waldron et al. (2001)
Motivational enhancement therapy (MET)/cognitive-behavioral therapy (CBT) 5 or 12 (MET/CBT)	Individual/ group	Youth ages 13–17; girls/ boys; outpatient/home	Dennis et al. (2004)
MET and motivational interviewing (MI)	Individual/ group	Youth ages 13–17	Tanner-Smith et al. (2013)
Multidimensional family therapy (MDFT)	Family	Youth ages 13–17; girls/ boys; outpatient/home	Liddle et al. (2009)
Multidimensional treatment foster care (MTFC)	Individual/ group family	Youth ages 13–17; MTFC foster home	Chamberlain & Reid (1998)
Multisystemic therapy (MST)	Brief individual	Youth ages 13–17; home, school, or community	Henggeler et al. (1999)
Parenting with Love and Limits (PLL)	Family	Youth ages 13–17	Smith et al. (2006)
Seeking Safety	Group or individual	Youth ages 13–17; outpatient, inpatient, residential	Najavits et al. (2006)
Seven Challenges® Program	Individual	Youth ages 13–17; outpatient	Stevens et al. (2007)
Teen Intervene	Individual	Youth ages 12–19; outpatient, school, or juvenile detention setting	Winters et al. (2012)

often include a motivational (interviewing) prelude to engagement and participation in more intensive treatment (e.g., CBT). Additional forms of BIs include its use as a substitute for more comprehensive treatment for persons seeking assistance but on waiting lists, and its use in primary care or other opportunistic settings such as schools or hospital emergency departments to facilitate referrals for additional specialized treatment (Tait & Hulse, 2003). The latter uses suggest its potential value as part of screening, brief intervention, and referral to treatment (SBIRT) programs.

Reviews have identified motivational interviewing (MI) techniques as a primary common component of most BIs in adolescents, perhaps because they can be delivered in multiple settings (e.g., primary care, emergency departments, schools) (Erickson, Gerstle, & Feldstein, 2005; Jensen et al., 2011; Tait & Hulse, 2003; Winters, Fahnhorst, Botzet, Lee, & Lalone, 2012). These are generally one to four sessions in duration and are usually based on MI principles (Mitchell, Gryczynski, O'Grady, & Schwartz, 2013). BIs are generally one-to-one sessions in duration and use feedback on substance use compared with norms (Erickson et al., 2005). These reviews also found that studies of the efficacy of BIs yielded mixed results. In some studies, the BI did not outperform a comparison condition, and yet for others, BIs showed significant efficacy (Tait & Hulse, 2003). BIs with adolescents generally show less reduction in alcohol use when compared with other drugs (Tait & Hulse, 2003). The strongest BI effects found in these studies tend to be related to harm reduction, such as reduction of substance-related driving and riding, alcohol-related injuries, unplanned sex, and other negative consequences of use. Effects on substance use have been more modest and tend to be stronger at shorter (<6 months) rather than longer follow-up intervals (>12 months).

New approaches to SBIRT have used computerized brief interventions. In a study of adolescents with self-reported alcohol use and aggressive behavior, multiple outcomes improved significantly 3 months after a computerized screening followed by a brief computerized or therapist-led intervention (Cunningham et al., 2009).

Family Therapies

A majority of the evidence-based models for the treatment of adolescents with SUDs involve family interventions. This is not surprising, as adolescents are usually dependent members of a family. The many family risk factors for the development and maintenance of problems substance use in adolescents also suggest family functioning as a primary target for intervention.

Based on the quality of the studies and replications in the field, two family-based approaches, functional family therapy (FFT) and multidimensional family therapy (MDFT), are well established for adolescent substance abuse treatment. Other family models, including multisystemic family therapy (MST), brief strategic family therapy (BSFT), and family behavior therapy (FBT), are probably efficacious, pending replications by independent research teams. Despite the collective evidence, however, no clear pattern emerged for the superiority of one treatment model over another.

Family interventions for substance abuse treatment have common goals: providing psychoeducation about SUDs, which decreases familial resistance to treatment and increases motivation and engagement; assisting parents and family to initiate and maintain efforts to get the adolescent into appropriate treatment and achieve abstinence; helping parents and family to establish or reestablish structure with consistent limit setting and careful monitoring of the adolescent's activities and behavior; improving communication among family members; and getting other family members into treatment and/or support programs. Specific engagement procedures have been incorporated as part of most family-based interventions.

Cognitive-Behavioral Therapies

Researchers have used several versions of CBT in clinical trials and some of these have manuals available outlining CBT for adolescent SUDs (see the Appendix). The CBT protocols are somewhat variable in length and do not all cover a complete set of topics. The most accessible version is from the Cannabis Youth Treatment (CYT) study (Diamond et al., 2002; SAMHSA, 2001), which consists of two versions in which individual sessions of motivational enhancement therapy (MET) precede group sessions of CBT. One version is MET/CBT 5 and the other is MET/CBT 12, with 5 and 12 sessions of CBT, respectively. The CYS did not show differences in outcome between the two versions; this suggests that briefer interventions are often effective, at least for this group of adolescents with mild to moderate severity of SUDs.

Contingency Management

Contingency management (CM) approaches using contingency contracting and vouchers also appear to be promising (Henggeler, Cunningham, & Rowland, 2011; Stanger & Budney, 2010). CM encompasses a variety of behaviorally oriented interventions, including motivational incentives as part of SUD treatment programs, as well as behavioral contracts and contingencies to reinforce abstinence and other behavioral changes at home.

Aftercare Interventions

SUDs are often chronic disorders requiring ongoing intervention. Naturalistic studies of adolescent SUD treatment find that attendance in aftercare treatment or self-support groups (e.g., Alcoholics Anonymous [AA] or Narcotics Anonymous [NA]) is related to positive outcomes (Kelly & Myers, 2007) and higher rates of abstinence and other measures of improved outcome when compared with adolescents not participating in such groups following treatment (Kelly et al., 2000).

Adolescents attending more intensive aftercare programs involving case management and community reinforcement were more likely than those who did not receive these services to be abstinent from marijuana and to reduce their alcohol use at 3 months postdischarge (Godley, Godley, Dennis, Funk, & Passetti, 2002). Empirical studies have found aftercare interventions for adolescents with SUDs to be efficacious (Godley, Godley, Dennis, Funk, & Passetti, 2007). After acute treatment for substance use, ongoing attention should be paid to comorbid psychopathology and other comprehensive needs of the adolescent and his or her family.

Twelve-Step Approaches

Twelve-step approaches have often been used as a basis for treatment. Attendance at AA and NA groups is an adjunct to professional treatment of SUDs. Twelve-step approaches, using AA and NA as a basis for treatment, are perhaps the most common approaches for treatment and treatment programs in the United States. As noted above, attendance in aftercare treatment or self-support groups (e.g., AA or NA) is related to positive outcomes in several studies of adolescent SUD treatment (Williams & Chang, 2000; Winters et al., 2000). Several other studies have found that attendance at self-help support or aftercare groups is associated with higher rates of abstinence and other measures of improved outcome when compared with those not participating in such groups after treatment (Brown, Myers, Mott, & Vik, 1994). Twelve-step programs can be defined as having adolescents work on specific steps toward recovery, attend self-support groups (AA or NA), and obtain the assistance of a sponsor who is another person in recovery from substance use problems.

PHARMACOLOGICAL TREATMENTS FOR SUDs

The majority of the research in pharmacotherapy of adolescents with SUDs relates to the treatment of comorbid psychiatric disorders, such as depression and ADHD. Strategies in pharmacological interventions for

SUDs include substitution therapies, detoxification, blocking therapies, craving reduction therapies, and aversion therapies (Bukstein & Horner, 2010).

Substitution therapies, which are used to prevent withdrawal, eliminate drug craving, and block the euphoric effects of illicit opiate use, use an agonist (e.g., nicotine replacement therapy [NRT] for nicotine dependence, methadone maintenance for opioid dependence) or a partial agonist (e.g., buprenorphine for opioid dependence) that acts on the same receptors that mediate the psychotropic effects of a substance.

Detoxification strategies generally use agonists or medications that provide symptomatic relief (e.g., clonidine for opioid withdrawal, benzodiazepines for alcohol withdrawal). In the absence of specific research, it is reasonable to use pharmacotherapy protocols for adolescents similar to those used in adults when needed. Aversive interventions, such as disulfiram (Antabuse), blocking strategies (e.g., naltrexone for opiate dependence), and anticraving medications (naltrexone, acamprosate, and ondansetron for alcohol; bupropion for nicotine; buprenorphine for opioids), require medication adherence and are likely most effective among patients with high motivation (Bukstein & Horner, 2010). Buprenorphine is a partial agonist. It is difficult to overdose on buprenorphine, and its combination with naloxone (opiate antagonist) makes it difficult to abuse intravenously. Naloxone is not absorbed orally and hence is not active if the combination is taken sublingually (buprenorphine alone is taken sublingually). If the combination medication is injected, naloxone blocks the opiate receptors and any euphoric effects of buprenorphine. Two double-blind placebo-controlled trials have demonstrated the efficacy of buprenorphine in retention in treatment and in reducing the number of positive urine tests for opiates compared to clonidine (Marsch et al., 2005) and fewer dropouts from maintenance treatment (Woody et al., 2008). With the possible exception of bupropion and buprenorphine, there is only very modest evidence supporting their use in adolescents. These agents should be prescribed to youth only after a thorough consideration of previous treatment attempts. Current evidence does not support use of pharmacotherapy for any other SUDs or other drug use (e.g., cocaine, stimulants, sedative/hypnotics, or club drugs) in adolescents.

N-Acetylcysteine (NAC) is a supplement presumed to affect glutamate modulation. Treatment-seeking cannabis-dependent adolescents who took NAC had more than twice the odds, compared with those receiving placebo, of having negative urine cannabinoid test results during treatment (Gray et al., 2012a).

Tobacco use or nicotine dependence is commonly present in adolescents with SUDs and/or psychiatric disorders, but few are diagnosed with nicotine dependence and offered smoking cessation treatment

(Upadhyaya, Deas, & Brady, 2005). NRTs (transdermal patch, gum, inhaler, and lozenge), varenicline, and bupropion sustained-release (SR) are currently approved by the U.S. Food and Drug Administration for smoking cessation in adults. NRT and bupropion SR are the agents most studied for adolescent smokers, with most studies of NRT using the transdermal nicotine patch. The efficacy of the transdermal nicotine patch and gum has been modest among adolescents, with resulting abstinence rates ranging from 5 to 18% (Moolchan et al., 2004). Nicotine withdrawal symptoms may be a significant problem in situations where adolescents with nicotine dependence cannot smoke, such as psychiatric hospitals, and NRT may need to be provided to counter nicotine withdrawal symptoms, even to non-treatment-seeking adolescent smokers (Upadhyaya et al., 2005). Bupropion has also shown promise in an open study (Upadhyaya, Brady, & Wang, 2004) and in a randomized controlled trial (Gray et al., 2011) in the treatment of adolescent smokers. In a randomized, blinded comparison of bupropion extended-release with varenicline, both agents improved nicotine abstinence, although no difference between the agents was reported (Gray, Carpenter, Lewis, Klintworth, & Upadhyaya, 2012b).

FROM EVIDENCE-BASED INTERVENTIONS TO PRACTICE

Knowledge of evidence-based approaches is important for clinicians. Certainly, formal training in one or more evidence-based practices for adolescents with SUDs provides clinicians with approaches on which they can build other clinical skills that can augment the proven efficacy of the evidence-based practice. Clinicians can also learn from the methods comprising the evidence-based practice and its component skills. This is the approach of the remaining chapters of this book: use of evidence-based approaches as the foundation for a clinician tool kit for dealing with youth having SUDs.

Almost all evidence-based practices for adolescents with SUDs were developed and tested with detailed protocols, often specifying specific inclusion and exclusion criteria and procedures for implementing the intervention/treatment practice. Clinicians do not have this luxury and must usually assess and treat each adolescent who walks through the door. Nevertheless, evidence-based practices offer a useful point of departure for the inevitable modification and changes that must accommodate community treatment of adolescents with SUDs, many of whom represent a much more difficult population of youth than those treated in clinical trials. While a number of detailed descriptions of these evidence-based interventions exist, more hands-on training and supervision in these procedures are recommended for delivery of these specific interventions. The clinician treating adolescents with SUDs can follow several general principles:

- Target motivation and engagement (see Chapter 2).
- Focus on skills for both the adolescent and his or her parents (see Chapters 6 and 7).
- Intervene with the family whenever possible (see Chapters 7 and 8).
- Deliver comprehensive services (e.g., obtaining education resources, housing, financial assistance) when needed.

The clinical directions presented in the remainder of this book are based on lessons learned during the practice of many of these evidence-based interventions, together with a heavy dose of clinical wisdom and experience, including critical aspects of these practices, gained from working with these youth for almost 30 years.

Chapter Two

Motivation and Engagement

Problems with motivation for SUD treatment are universal—so much so that denial (i.e., "I really don't have a problem") is considered one of the primary psychological symptoms of addiction. Poor motivation, or no motivation at all, is especially prominent in adolescents with SUDs. While the importance of denial in SUDs is beyond dispute, poor motivation is determined by many factors. For adolescents, immature cognitive control (see Chapter 1), poor insight, strong desire for autonomy, and frequent presence of an oppositional–defiant behavioral pattern often result in a lack of desire for treatment. This opposition relates to a general resistance to any adult demand for change. However, it doesn't always indicate the adolescent's overall measure of motivation to change a specific behavior. In addition, developmental deficits in executive functioning often result in poor problem recognition. Regardless, few adolescents either present themselves for treatment or go willingly without some level of protest. This might take the form of behavioral action (e.g., arguing, running away) or passivity (e.g., not talking during assessment or frequently responding "I don't know").

Many in the field insist that "denial" must be broken or confronted before treatment can commence or be successful. In traditional treatment settings, this might take the form of confrontation in which the professional provides direct, "reality-oriented" feedback to a client regarding the client's own thoughts, feelings, or behavior. Despite the sincerity and concern of such professionals, confrontational communications may range from frank feedback to anger-tinged, profanity-laden indictments, denunciations of character, challenges and ultimatums, intense argumentation, ridicule, and humiliation. In group settings, such confrontation often comes from peers. Despite the absence of evidence that confrontational strategies work for either adults or adolescents in SUD treatment, well-meaning professionals or peers in treatment often frame resistance to confrontation as "denial" and blame the patient for not willingly accepting this feedback. They may believe the teen needs to "hit bottom" before "accepting" the need for treatment.

An adolescent's motivation for treatment is not something that requires tearing down but rather building up. Enhancing motivation is a routine part of treatment and an important skill for professionals dealing with adolescents. Motivational engagement is important in promoting an accurate, truthful account of the adolescent's behaviors. Motivational strategies are important in assessment, extend into treatment, and should be considered for both the adolescent and the parent.

To establish a therapeutic relationship that promotes motivation, engaging with the teenager and his parents is critical. Engagement advances trust and trust advances hope. Where there is hope, adolescents and parents can begin to believe in change and to recognize that change is possible. Belief or self-efficacy is often an essential ingredient, which, in addition to motivation, leads to behavioral change.

I begin this chapter by discussing general motivational and engagement issues concerning parents and families. Next, I explore the issue of coercion and whether it can ever be appropriate. I then focus on two sets of evidence-based strategies used to enhance motivation for treatment: (1) motivational interviewing (MI) and (2) contingency management (CM). MI and CM are not mutually exclusive. In most cases, a clinician should use some aspects of each in any attempt to optimize motivation for treatment and treatment compliance.

PARENT AND FAMILY MOTIVATION AND ENGAGEMENT

Motivation of parents and other family members is highly relevant to the success of adolescents treated for SUDs. Treatment cannot progress unless parents or key family members are engaged and actively participate in the treatment process, helping to define problems, setting goals, and implementing interventions to meet those goals. The content of therapy, regardless of how potentially valuable it may be, will usually have little effect in the absence of a strong therapeutic alliance. Family members who are not engaged in treatment are unlikely to put forth the effort needed for favorable outcomes.

What are the keys to establishing and maintaining engagement? Empathy on behalf of the clinician is a precondition for client and family engagement, cutting across schools of psychotherapy. Empathy starts with therapist knowledge and confidence that he or she can help the family. If the family believes that the clinician is confident, they will believe that they can change and solve their problems at home, which increases their sense of self-efficacy. When the family feels more hopeful and finds that they have improved skills after clinical sessions, they become more engaged in treatment. The clinician creates an atmosphere of problem solving, respect, and choice.

Empathy requires demonstration of an understanding of expectations, family-generated goals, obstacles to treatment, and cultural considerations. Lack of empathy is a critical barrier to engagement and treatment success. Other obstacles reflect familial, adolescent, or other environmental issues and should be identified and targeted. Several proximal parent influences on the engagement process include SUDs, mental health problems (e.g., untreated parental bipolar disorder), intellectual limitations, level of comfort with receiving services (embarrassment), extent of suffering, and poor self-efficacy expectations (doubts that personal behavior can produce favorable outcomes).

More distal influences on the engagement process include family factors such as low parental bonding with the child (why engage if the child isn't liked or loved?); marital conflicts regarding treatment; extrafamilial influences such as employment status; social isolation (low social supports); a history of coercive or adversarial interactions with mental health or social service providers (children had previously been removed from the home by social welfare); and secondary gain associated with the status quo (the financial benefits of having a child with a disability). Environmental factors influencing engagement may also result from referral processes such as how much choice parents have about receiving services (e.g., is it a condition of probation for the child?), how treatment was presented to the family, and outcome expectations generated by the referral sources. Clinicians need to assess and address these factors and their potential influence on treatment success. At a minimum, clinicians should explore parent motivation(s) for having their adolescent in treatment, their goals and expectations for treatment, and their expectation for their level of active participation in treatment. Some parents may feel it is the clinician's job to change their teen, not theirs, and that they only need to bring the adolescent to treatment and pay for it. Questions to ask parents include the following:

"What would you like (or expect) to happen as a result of being here today?"
"What are your goals for treatment?"
"What do you think you will need to do for your adolescent to get better?"
"Do you think this treatment will work?"

Finally, self-efficacy on the part of parent(s) is critical. No doubt, parents may feel they have failed up to this point. Most parents try to use a variety of methods to promote change in their teen's behavior, including punishment, bribing, and/or ignoring, and see little, if any, improvement. Parents often carry substantial levels of hopelessness about this situation and their ability to remedy their adolescent's problems. Because clinicians are recognized as experts, parents often expect them to have the knowledge, skills, and resources necessary to solve the family's current difficulties because they, the parents, do not. Failing skills and competencies, low empowerment, and a history of interpersonal ineffectiveness often demoralize parents to the point that they feel incapable of effecting desired change or may be incapable of achieving outcomes in their present state (e.g., being depressed and/or cocaine abusing). Such characteristics in parents can generate a host of negative affective responses during the initial stages of therapy, for both the parent and the practitioner, and present significant challenges for the evolving therapeutic relationship. Grasping the underlying bases of demoralization allows the clinician to develop strategies to address those specific contributors.

Cognitive factors such as parent and adolescent beliefs, expectations, attributions, and perceptions often contribute to engagement and resistance to specific interventions (Robin & Foster, 1989). Unreasonable parent beliefs about the teen can include: (1) *malicious intent* (the adolescent's behavior *always* reflects a desire to hurt, annoy, or anger parents), (2) *ruination* (if the adolescent is given freedom, it will ruin his or her future), (3) *obedience* (the adolescent should *always* do what his or her parents ask), (4) *perfectionism* (the adolescent should *always* make the right decisions and do the right thing), (5) *love and appreciation* (the adolescent should *always* appreciate everything his or her parents do for him or her), and (6) *self-blame* (the parents blame *all* the adolescent's problems on their own failings and mistakes). Similar unreasonable adolescent beliefs include (1) *ruination* (the adolescent's life will be ruined by his or her parents' rules), (2) *fairness* (it is unfair for the adolescent to have rules), and (3) *autonomy* (the adolescent should not have to follow any rules and instead should be granted absolute freedom).

Life is more complex, however. Rigid adherence to these unreasonable beliefs by parents and/or adolescents may interfere with clinician attempts to change parental behavior, which requires acknowledgment of some level of adolescent autonomy and the likelihood that the adolescent's recovery from SUDs will not be perfect. In addition, the teen is typically going to be unwilling to accept any limits on his or her behavior. In Chapters 6 and 7, I will discuss how the clinician addresses such unreasonable adolescent and parent beliefs.

In practice, engagement requires soliciting both the parent's and the adolescent's concerns and goals, if any. A willingness to listen to both sides of the family's story and to facilitate communication of each family member's perception and concerns assists this engagement. Treatment is often taken up with overcoming barriers. Attempts to target these barriers should be made within a context that is generally conducive to engagement. Essential components of effective engagement include the quality of the interaction, the collaborative nature of developing tasks and goals of treatment, and the personal bond between the adolescent and his or her family (specifically parents) and the clinician. To begin with, the clinician should explain the rationale, possible benefits, and structure of treatment. In addition, he or she should identify family strengths and use a collaborative approach with the family, seeing family members as full partners in the treatment process. The clinician might say: "What are your concerns? What can I do to help *you?*"

Additional engagement strategies are discussed later in this chapter under Motivational Interviewing and in Chapter 3 on assessment.

Is Coercion Ever Appropriate?

Many in the SUD treatment community have argued that little benefit can be derived when a substance user is forced into treatment, either by the criminal justice system, by parents, or, in some cases, by schools. Some oppose coerced treatment on philosophical grounds. Others argue against it on clinical grounds, maintaining that treatment can be effective only if the person is truly motivated to change. A variation of this position is that addicts must "hit bottom" before they are able to benefit from treatment, a circumstance that is not necessarily true of most coerced clients. According to this view, it is a poor investment to devote time and resources to adolescents who are unlikely to change because they have little or no motivation to change their behaviors related to substance use.

Broadly defined, coercion refers to the imposition of treatment over the adolescent's objections or regardless of the adolescent's preferences, which can be considered an infringement of autonomy. Coercion can be a legal mandate, such as civil commitment, court-ordered treatment, and diversion-to-treatment programs (drug courts). Formal nonlegal coercion includes mandatory referrals to treatment by schools; coercion can also take the form of informal social pressure (threats) by parents, other family members, and friends. Most of these forms of coercion serve as a means of initiating treatment. In traditional programs, coercive behavior often involves use of confrontational communications (such as those listed in the beginning of this chapter). However, the use of confrontation, threats, and attempts at intimidation by those trying to get adolescents into treatment or by clinicians during treatment is counterproductive and generally increases resistance to treatment. Some parents utilize an extralegal means of forcing their adolescent children into residential treatment by employing third parties to forcibly escort the teens to treatment facilities, which are often located in a remote part of the country. There have been reports of adolescents being forcibly detained at some of these centers. Such extreme measures are often counterproductive and have the potential for physical and emotional harm. Delegating extralegal coercion to others serves to reinforce parental impotence. These types of coercive communication should be eliminated from the treatment of adolescents.

At the same time, research shows that legal mandates and other nonlegal sanctions do not result in worse outcomes and may improve outcomes by keeping youth in treatment longer; I recommend their judicious use. Examples of nonlegal coercion include contingencies (or consequences) imposed by parents or others such as schools. These consequences include alternative school placements and loss of privileges (e.g., no cell phones, no video games, and/or grounding). For example, coercion by the juvenile justice system is one of the most common methods for entering adolescents into treatment. Treatment is either court-ordered in the case of adjudicated youth or "highly recommended" for youth threatened with adjudication. In addition to traditional adjudication—or threat of adjudication—as a delinquent, juvenile justice officials across the United States are embracing a new method of dealing with adolescent substance abuse. Importing a popular innovation from adult courts, state and local governments have started hundreds of specialized drug courts to provide judicial supervision and to coordinate substance abuse treatment for drug-involved juveniles.

Drug courts give offenders an opportunity to change their behavior and to stop their use of illegal drugs before they receive serious legal penalties. Those who stop using drugs and complete a rigorous program of treatment may have their charges dismissed or their sentences reduced. To ensure that program adolescents complete drug treatment as ordered, drug courts often assume responsibilities that go beyond the traditional role of a criminal court. Many drug courts coordinate client case management and probation supervision for every case. They hold regular review meetings with the youth and his or her family as well as frequent court hearings to monitor each offender's situation. They use graduated sanctions and tangible rewards to motivate offender compliance with treatment, and they check for violations by conducting numerous random or unannounced drug tests. Immediate sanctions in the form of detention or other placement are made upon violation of drug court stipulations of compliance with treatment and/or substance use.

A number of states have involuntary commitment laws that apply to adolescents with SUDs. These laws require parents or another responsible party such as a physician to file with a local court. Following a court-approved evaluation, a recommendation for treatment—usually for residential treatment—may be forwarded to a judge or his or her representative. These commitments are in many ways similar to the procedures involved in drug courts or in delinquency adjudications, although the adolescent need not have committed a crime to qualify. In many of these instances, provisions for monitoring are difficult. For example, since this is usually outside the formal juvenile justice system, there is no probation officer to do drug testing to monitor compliance. Compliance is also generally defined as treatment attendance rather than abstinence.

When an adolescent enters treatment because of a legal mandate or other type of coercion, the professional will likely be faced with noncooperation. The strategies of MI offer ways to respond productively.

MOTIVATIONAL INTERVIEWING

Owing to normal developmental concerns such as the search for autonomy, adolescents tend to mistrust clinicians, often throughout the therapy, and they show this mistrust through crude, intense, and provocative behavior. Therapists need to prepare for it. Many clinicians, like parents, may be tempted to address adolescents' "resistance" with aggressive confrontation, resulting in a power struggle and an emotional shouting match. The harder the clinician pushes to resolve the problem, the worse the situation becomes. Not surprisingly, a confrontational style of counseling often leads to resistance in adolescents who feel their personal freedom or autonomy is threatened. Yet, when adolescents feel that they are choosing to do something in their own self-interest, their motivation can be intense. MI is an approach that accounts for the inherent ambivalence in adolescents about changing their behavior (Miller & Rollnick, 2013).

MI is defined by its developers, William R. Miller and Stephen Rollnick (2013) as a directive, client-centered counseling style for eliciting behavior change by helping clients to explore and resolve ambivalence. Examining and resolving the ambivalence is the central purpose of MI. Although a number of variations, adaptations, and techniques are used under the umbrella of MI (e.g., MET, motivational enhancement therapy, a type of expanded MI), these are all grounded by a set of guiding principles called the "spirit" of MI. The core elements include the following:

1. MI is a particular kind of *conversation about change*.
2. MI is *collaborative* (a person-centered partnership between the clinician and adolescent [or parent] that honors autonomy, but not an "expert–recipient" relationship).
3. MI is *evocative* in that it seeks to promote the person's own motivation and commitment.

MI requires training and practice. In this introduction to MI (a full discussion of its elements and practice is beyond the scope of this book), I discuss the four fundamental processes of MI and some specific techniques for eliciting the processes in treating adolescents with SUDs. The four fundamental processes—engaging, guiding, evoking, and planning—generally occur consecutively, but overall they are rarely linear, and clinicians will continue to use engagement techniques while proceeding with guiding, evoking, and planning. Throughout the processes, clinicians use techniques to express empathy, develop discrepancy, roll with resistance, and support self-efficacy. A key objective is for the clinician to listen for and reflect back "change talk." Change talk is any adolescent speech that favors movement in the direction of change. Conversely, any adolescent speech that goes toward maintaining the status quo is labeled "sustain talk."

Engaging

Engaging is a relational process whose primary goal is to establish empathy, that is, an understanding of the adolescent's perception of his or her problem(s). Establishing empathy is achieved through the use of skills known by the acronym of OARS: open-ended questions, affirmations, reflections, and summaries. Although OARS are most often associated with establishing empathy at the beginning of the clinician–adolescent relationship, they can be used throughout the course of a session and for the duration of treatment. The skills are used strategically to promote discussion of some topics while minimizing the discussion of others. Acceptance facilitates change, while pressure to change elicits resistance. An atmosphere of safety promotes self-focus and self-disclosure. For the adolescent who is used to others trying to tell him or her what to do, such a stance can be disarming. The following section describes the benefits and characteristics of each OARS skill.

Open-Ended Questions

- Open-ended questions can be answered with a wide range of responses. They offer the adolescent choice in how to respond.
- These questions seek information, invite the client's perspective, or encourage elaboration and self-exploration.
- They encourage the client to do most of the talking.

> "Tell me about your marijuana use. . . ."
>
> "How have you been doing with cutting down on your marijuana use?"

Affirmations

■ Affirmations provide support and enhance rapport.

■ They complement and may be statements of appreciation, understanding, or acknowledgment of strengths.

> "It must have been hard to come in here and talk with me about this."
> "That's a good suggestion."
> "You're a very resourceful person to use so much and not to get into any trouble."
> "When you set your mind to something, you do it."

Reflective Listening

■ Reflective listening conveys to the adolescent that you have heard what was said and understand.

■ It serves as a check on the meaning of the adolescent's statements and/or the feelings behind them.

■ Types of reflections include:

□ Simple repetition (of what the adolescent said).

□ Substitution of words with the same meaning (paraphrasing).

□ Reflection of meaning (the clinician states what he or she feels is the meaning of the adolescent's statement).

□ Reflection of emotion (the clinician states what he or she believes the adolescent is feeling).

□ Amplified reflection: Only the negative side of ambivalence is reflected.

□ Double-sided reflection: Both sides of ambivalence are reflected.

□ Continuing the paragraph (reflection plus addition of what the clinician thinks the adolescent might say next).

For example, the adolescent might say:

> "My parents are always on my case about getting high. They search my room for my supply, they listen in on my phone calls, and they sometimes even follow me when I go out."

Possible clinician reflections include:

■ *Using simple reflection* (saying what the client has said but in different words):
> "They bug you about smoking marijuana, and they spy on you about it."

- *Using reflection of meaning* (restating the meaning that may be implied by the words):
  "As though they're always trying to figure out if and when you're getting high."
- *Using reflection of feeling* (restating what you perceive to be the feeling conveyed in the client's statement):
  "It sounds like it's annoying to you, for them to get on your case like that."
- *Using amplified reflection:*
  "Your parents are really mean; they never give you a break."

Overstating as well as understating tends to cause adolescents to continue exploring and tell you more.

- *Using double-sided reflection:*
  "Your parents don't trust you and give you a hard time, but it sounds like they are concerned about your marijuana use."
  "On the one hand, you want to keep getting high, but you'd also like to get your mom off your back."
- *Continuing the paragraph:*
  "Your parents bug you way too much . . . it's really none of their business, and they need to let you make your own decisions and live your own life."

Summaries

A summary is a *reflection* that draws together content from two or more prior client statements. There are different types of summaries:

- *Collecting summary:* Draws together comments or change talk and invites continued talk. For example:
  "So far you have told me how your parents invade your privacy and otherwise interfere with your life, and you are angry about that. You do not think they care about you anyway. You would not want to stop your marijuana use for them."
- *Linking summary:* Ties together current and previously said ideas to encourage reflection of relationship between concepts. For example:

  ADOLESCENT: My parents are always bothering me about my grades and the friends I hang with.

  CLINICIAN: You feel that your parents are giving you a hard time. But you also mentioned before that trouble caused by your marijuana use was getting in the way of your job and some of your relationships.

- *Transitional summary:* Marks and announces shift of topic. For example:
  "Talking about your marijuana use gets you angry with your parents and school bothering you. They think you aren't doing well because of using. They invade your privacy. It all makes you angry, even depressed. You are more concerned about those feelings and how to deal with your anger."

Rolling with Resistance

Even more than adults with SUDs, adolescents often display resistance to changing their behavior. In using MI with adolescents, one finds perhaps the most value through the use of strategies to handle resistance. Miller and Rollnick (2013) described four types of resistance: (1) arguing—the adolescent challenges, discounts, or is hostile to the clinician; (2) interrupting—the adolescent cuts the clinician off or talks over him or her; (3) denying—the adolescent blames others, minimizes, disagrees, makes excuses, and is reluctant; and (4) ignoring—the adolescent is inattentive and does not respond or give input. A fifth type of resistance is lack of compliance—the adolescent does not show up, misses, or frequently cancels sessions.

A goal of MI is to reduce resistance because a lower level of adolescent resistance is associated with long-term change. MI offers clinicians specific approaches to addressing resistance. Resistance is viewed not as an adolescent trait but as a normal response to a perceived threat in an interpersonal context. Resistance communicates to the clinician that the clinician is moving too fast and needs to appropriately match the adolescent. Defusing resistance requires clinicians to change their approach and increase the adolescent's sense of control by using the following strategies:

- *Shifting focus:* Talk about another topic but one less likely to provoke a resistant response.
- *Emphasizing personal choice and control:* Agree or remind adolescents that you cannot make decisions for them or force them to do something they really do not wish to do.
- *Reframing:* Invite the client to consider a different interpretation of what has been said.
- *Agreement with a twist:* Focus on *reflection* or *affirmation,* or accord followed by a reframe.
- *Coming alongside:* Accept and reflect the client's theme.

Examples of some of these strategies follow.

> ADOLESCENT: I don't have to be here. You can't make me go to rehab! I told my parents that I am not quitting smoking.
>
> CLINICIAN: You are right; I cannot make you do anything. [emphasizing personal choice/control] But I appreciate your being here today. Given how you must feel, it must have taken a lot of effort to come.
>
> ADOLESCENT: I guess. But my parents—they are always on my case.
>
> CLINICIAN: They—your parents—have no reason to give you a hard time. You may use, but it's not causing *any* problems for you. [coming alongside]
>
> ADOLESCENT: Well, I wouldn't say that—I got caught with weed at school.
>
> CLINICIAN: But your folks are really complaining too much, but maybe there are some downsides to using weed? [agreement with a twist]

Guiding

In the strategic process of guiding, the primary goals are agenda setting and finding a strategic focus of the interaction between clinician and adolescent. The clinician assists the adolescent in examining his or her goals and values and in finding any perceived discrepancy between present behavior and important goals or values (i.e., the discrepancy between where I am and where I want to be or who I am and who I want to be). The adolescent's experience of discrepancy enhances the importance of change. An awareness of consequences is crucial, and objective information through feedback serves to provide this awareness. In the end, the adolescent should present the arguments for change. In finding a change goal or in setting an agenda, the clinician helps the teen to focus on one behavior that the adolescent agrees to target. Nevertheless, the clinician needs to understand the adolescent's agenda while being open and honest about the goals of treatment. For example, the adolescent may point to school or parent problems or depressive symptoms as his change goal, while the clinician may realize that substance use should be the target. Through the use of selective OARS responses, the clinician may guide the adolescent to reasonable consideration of other goals, such as decreasing substance use behavior. Because multiple problems may benefit from change, the clinician helps the patient select a behavior to discuss.

ADOLESCENT: I am not ready to quit using and no one can make me.

CLINICIAN: True, It's likely that no one can make you stop. I appreciate your honesty and willingness to talk about what's going on in your life. You made it clear that you do not want to stop using marijuana, but you have reported that you could cut down or not use in dangerous situations such as driving. You also said that you are often anxious or angry. We could focus on these problems—what's important to you.

The technique most closely associated with this phase is decisional balance (see Figure 2.1). In this technique, the clinician maintains a neutral but curious stance while guiding the teen to consider the pros and cons of both changing and not changing. Similarly, providing information or advice (see Table 2.2 on p. 35) to the adolescent is often useful not only in this phase but throughout MI. But providing information and advice must be done carefully in the MI spirit to avoid violating the collaborative aspect of the clinician–adolescent interaction. Before providing information or advice, the clinician should almost always ask permission or await an invitation, with frequent qualifications that the adolescent should make the decision.

Finally, when the clinician feels that the adolescent has reached an outcome, this should be explicitly summarized in the following ways: either

Goal: consider both pros and cons of change versus no change

Example: continued marijuana use

	Changing	Not Changing
Benefits/Pros	Fewer school problems Get along with parents better Not late to or skip work so much	Get high Hang out with using friends Feel more relaxed
Costs/Cons	Lose using friends More bored	Get into trouble more More school problems Feel lousy when using too much

FIGURE 2.1. Decisional balance.

the adolescent is not interested in changing any behavior; the adolescent is willing to talk further about changing his or her behavior; or the adolescent is ambivalent. This summary is not the end, for it might further the discussion. The clinician always emphasizes adolescent autonomy: *It's really up to you to decide when or if you want to make any changes.* While the adolescent usually presents a goal for change, occasionally he or she will select none of the above options, indicating a lack of any interest. If the clinician accepts the MI philosophy, he or she must accept the adolescent's decision and not press or confront the teenager.

Supporting Self-Efficacy

Self-efficacy is another important element that the clinician seeks to bolster in the adolescent. Motivation or a willingness to change is often not the main obstacle, but rather the adolescent often lacks self-efficacy (the confidence that one can succeed at a task) or readiness (an appreciation of the importance of change now rather than sometime in the future). The readiness/importance rule (see Figure 2.2) can be used to measure the extent to which the adolescent might be ready for change now. Assuming the teen is ready for change, the same rule can be used to measure how confident he or she is in the ability to change. Similarly, tracking change talk can give the clinician an idea of how ready and able the adolescent is for change. For self-efficacy and confidence, this means following and evoking confidence talk through the following techniques:

- Elaboration: "Tell me more about . . ."
- Scaling confidence/confidence ruler (see Figure 2.2).
- Reviewing successes: "You mentioned that you quit for more than 6 months a while ago."
- Personal strengths and supports: "You said you had some friends who wanted to help you—would that make a difference?"
- Brainstorming: "Let's try to think of some successes that you have had."
- Information and advice: "If it's OK with you, I think I know of some reasons you might be able to succeed."
- Reframing failures: "It sounds like you learned a lot about relapses."
- Hypothetical change: "Can you imagine what your life would be like if you stopped using?"

We have discussed several of these techniques previously. Hypothetical change is similar to envisioning and asks the adolescent to think of what change in the behavior—and no change—will be like in the future. Reviewing successes and reframing failure ("learning experiences") can

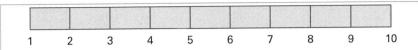

- Using the ruler shown above, the adolescent indicates how ready or confident he or she is to make a change (quit or cut down) to specific drug use (or all drug use).
- If the adolescent is not at all ready to make a change, he or she would circle the 1. If he or she is extremely ready or confident to make a change, he or she would circle the 10. If he or she is unsure whether to make a change, he or she would circle 3, 4, or 5.
- Rate importance/readiness and confidence separately on the same above scale.
- If the adolescent rates him- or herself high, ask why. This elicits change talk since the client will give reasons that he or she is ready and/or confident about change.
- If the adolescent rates him- or herself low, ask why he or she is not higher and/or what it would take for the client to rate him- or herself higher.

FIGURE 2.2. Importance/readiness scale and confidence scale.

add much to an adolescent's self-efficacy and confidence to change. Brain-storming, as a collaborative exercise, allows the clinician and adolescent to work together to consider change options that might be more accept-able to the adolescent and that the adolescent feels capable of completing successfully.

Evoking

Evoking refers to the clinician task of getting the adolescent to talk more about change. Evoking provides the bridge to change once a clear change goal has been set. The clinician continues to use OARS selectively while paying attention to perhaps the best metric for motivation and intention for change—change talk. The clinician attempts not only to recognize change talk but also to elicit it (e.g., through use of selective questions), responds to change talk (e.g., through use of selective reflections), and summarizes change talk. For example:

"You have made it clear that you do not wish to stop, but you have also reported other problems such as using in a safe place and having mood changes and anxiety."
"What would you like to do?"
"Where do we go from here?"
"What now?"

Types of change talk include (1) preparatory change talk, (2) confidence talk, and (3) implementing talk. Preparatory change talk expresses motivations for change without stating specific intent or commitment to change. It includes adolescent discussion of the disadvantages of the status quo, problem recognition, and concern, as well as speech about the advantages of change. Miller and Rollnick (2013) use the acronym DARN—desire, ability, reason, and need—to describe the type of expressions that convey preparatory or confidence talk. A fifth category, commitment, extends DARN to include most types of change talk and expresses the intention to change. Implementing talk represents the resolution of ambivalence and includes statements indicating not only willingness but also ability, readiness, preparation, and commitment to take steps to change.

Commitment and intention are the best verbal predictors of actual change in the adult MI literature. Confidence talk indicates the adolescent's perceived ability to change manifested by such statements as "I can change" or specifically, "I can stop using. . . ."

- Desire: "I really want to quit. I wish I did not use so much."
- Ability: "I think I can cut down on my marijuana use."
- Reason: "If I want to finish high school, I have to stop drinking on weeknights."
- Need: "I have to stop."
- Commitment: "I am going to cut down—maybe stop."

Evoking Change Talk

- Evocative questions (also see above).
    "What do you think you are going to do?"
    "What does all this mean?"
    "What do you think has to change?"
    "What are your options now?"
    "Where do we go from here?"
    "How are you going to deal with this?"
    "What's the next step?"
    "It sounds like you are ready to stop using. . . . ?"
    "What makes you willing to stop using. . . . ?"
    "Sounds like you are considering a change. . . . ?"
- Elaboration.
    "Tell me more."
    "Give me some examples."

- Typical periods.
  "Tell me about a typical week or day of your marijuana use."
- Looking forward—if things don't change:
  "What if you don't stop?"
  "What if you do not change?"
  "What would be different?"
  "What would like be like in 5, 10 years from now?"
- Looking back.
  "How were things different before you started using . . . ?"
- Using extremes.
  "What is the worst thing (scenario) that might happen if you do not make a change?"
  "What is the best thing (scenario) if you do make a change?"
- Exploring goals and values.
  "How does using jibe with your goals?"
- Decisional balance (see Figure 2.1).
- Scaling importance/readiness and confidence (see Figure 2.2).

Table 2.1 summarizes methods of evoking change talk and confidence talk.

Responding to change talk is also critical to keep the adolescent talking about change. Using another acronym, EARS, the clinician solicits more change talk by elaborating (more detail, examples), affirming (positive comments about the adolescent's change talk), reflecting, and summarizing (a variation on the use of OARS). Recapitulation, a specific type of grand summary, strives to summarize and check the adolescent's perception of his or her problems (e.g., ambivalence, evidence of risks, intention to change) and the adolescent's situation from the clinician's perspective.

> CLINICIAN: So, from our conversation so far, you say that you have a school suspension—maybe even expulsion—hanging over you. You may have to go to juvenile court. And that's not counting how much grief your parents give you about smoking marijuana. But you like the way marijuana makes you feel—relaxed, deals with stress and most of your friends use too. What now? Where do you go from here? [summary followed by evocative question]
>
> ADOLESCENT: I am not sure. I wish my life was better. I want to do better and not get into trouble. [desire to change]

TABLE 2.1. Motivational Strategies

Methods that evoke change talk

- Evocative questions: strategic open questions the natural answer to which is change talk.
- Elaboration: an interviewer response to client change talk, asking for additional detail, clarification, or example.
- Typical periods: asking for usual times involving the behavior being changed.
- Looking forward: a strategy for evoking client change talk, exploring a possibly better future that the client hopes for or imagines, or anticipating the future consequences of not changing.
- Looking back: a strategy for evoking client change talk, exploring a better time in the past.
- Using extremes: exaggerating client statements in order to get clarification.
- Exploring goals and values: a strategy for evoking change talk by having people describe their most important life goals or values.
- Decisional balance: a choice-focused technique that can be used when counseling with neutrality, devoting equal exploration to the pros and cons of change or of a specific plan.
- Scaling importance: use of 1–10 scale to determine how important change is to the client, why change is important, or what keeps the change from being more important.

Methods that evoke confidence talk

- Evocative questions.
- Elaboration.
- Scaling confidence: use of a 1–10 scale to determine how confident the client is that he or she can change, why he or she is confident, or what keeps him or her from being more confident.
- Reviewing successes: listing areas where the client has experienced success.
- Personal strengths and supports: Listing available resources for support.
- Brainstorming: generating options without initially critiquing them.
- Information and advice: when the clinician provides information about change or advice about change; must occur only after permission or request from client.
- Reframing failures: an interviewer statement that invites the client to consider a different interpretation of what has been said.
- Hypothetical change: asking the client to imagine a particular change in behavior and possible results.

CLINICIAN: What do you see in the future if you don't make these changes? [looking forward]

ADOLESCENT: I probably won't finish high school and I'll probably end up in juvenile detention.

CLINICIAN: And if you do change?

ADOLESCENT: I think I would like to go to college. If I was still using, I would probably never go to class. [reasons]

CLINICIAN: Anything else that would be possible if you make a change?

ADOLESCENT: I could probably keep a boyfriend—and a job. [reasons]

CLINICIAN: So completing high school, going to college, keeping a job and boyfriend are important to you? Maybe more important than using? [exploring values/goals]

ADOLESCENT: I think I can do this—cut down or even stop if I need to. I can't keep getting into trouble. [need to change; reasons for change]

Being Ready for Change

Despite the willingness to change and confidence that change could occur, the adolescent has to be ready for change; that is, he or she thinks that change is important now. Change talk that indicates readiness/importance is often found in statements indicating a need to change ("I have to quit soon or I am going to detention") or implementing talk ("I am going to talk with the school counselor tomorrow"). Table 2.2 lists indicators that can help clinicians recognize readiness to change in an adolescent. In attempting to move the adolescent toward readiness/importance, the clinician can use the readiness/importance scale (Figure 2.2) and/

TABLE 2.2. Recognizing Readiness to Change

- Showing decreased resistance.
- Showing cooperation and collaboration.
- Asking fewer questions about the problem.
- Asking more questions about solutions and change.
- Making spontaneous change talk.
- Expressing resolve.
- Envisioning solution or change.
- Experimenting: showing willingness to try methods toward change.

or decisional balance (Figure 2.1) regarding a decision to make a change (stop using or enter treatment) now as opposed to later. Using the spirit of MI, the adolescent recognizes that the decision is his or hers to make. The clinician guides the discussion.

Planning

Planning is the final and perhaps most important step toward change, through which the clinician negotiates change goals and develops a specific change plan (see Table 2.3). In addition, the clinician seeks to strengthen the adolescent's commitment to change while managing implementation of the plan, including any ongoing adjustment of the plan.

The clinician should attempt to get the adolescent to be as specific as possible in identifying the elements of the plan. Writing the change plan down is highly recommended. First, the adolescent makes a clear statement of the goals of the plan (e.g., cut down or stop use, do better in school, get along better with parents or peers). Second, he or she restates the reasons for change, which serves to remind the teen of the specific motivation for change. Third, the adolescent lists specific steps toward change, both what he or she will do and when he or she will do it (e.g., "I will go to outpatient treatment"; "I will avoid using friends"). It is important to list supports (parents/peers/others) and potential obstacles (cues, substance availability), including the adolescent's planned response(s) to those obstacles. Finally, the clinician should inquire about signs of progress and success. How will the teen know when he or she is getting closer to the stated goals?

TABLE 2.3. Elements of a Change Plan

- Setting goals.
- Summarizing reasons for change.
- Considering change options.
- Arriving at a plan.
  - Steps: What will the client do and when?
  - Support: Who will be there for support of change, and how will they provide the support?
  - Obstacles: Anticipate obstacles and how they will be overcome.
  - Signs of progress: How will the client identify that what he or she is doing is working and goals are being met?
- Eliciting commitment: "Do you think that you can do this?"
                        "Is this something you want to do?"

"It looks like you are really committed to change. Do you know how you will do this? Perhaps the best way to get this done is to write up a change plan."

Development of a change plan often involves negotiation. The clinician should elicit options for goals and for the steps for change from the adolescent and should prompt a review of the options for adolescent preferences and self-efficacy. Many adolescents offer shoulder shrugs rather than specifics, showing their need for assistance in coming up with options. Such help constitutes advice, and so the clinician needs to ask permission.

CLINICIAN: If it's OK with you, I can review some change goals and treatment options that adolescents find useful? What do you think?

ADOLESCENT: I don't know how to do this.

CLINICIAN: Let's create a problem list, based on what you have told me. Let's start with improving your mood—that's number one according to your report. Then controlling anxiety. Getting along better with your mother. Then you did say that cutting down on your marijuana use was something that would help you. Any ideas on how you—or we—can tackle these problems?

ADOLESCENT: I am not sure how to do this?

CLINICIAN: If it's all right, I can tell you some of the ways that have helped other kids like you?

ADOLESCENT: Sure.

CLINICIAN: One way is meeting with a counselor—maybe me. Another way is to meet with a group of other kids with similar problems. Still another way is to meet with a counselor and your parents. Or you could do a little of all of these. What do you think?

ADOLESCENT: Maybe a group. I know my friends have these problems, and sometimes it helps to talk about them with other kids my age.

CLINICIAN: So, we decide to start with a group. We have a group that meets several times a week. Do you think you can and will attend? What are obstacles to your getting to these groups—or staying in group?

ADOLESCENT: Well, sometimes, I lose motivation—I'd rather hang out in my room.

CLINICIAN: Well, sometimes we ask parents to kick in extra privileges if kids come to treatment and are cooperative. We also have a kind of lottery at the group that gives prizes if you come to treatment.

ADOLESCENT: That might work.

CLINICIAN: I have written this down: you're going to groups with other kids, you're going to work on improving your mood and reducing your anxiety, and cutting down on your marijuana use, especially in risky situations? Agreed?

ADOLESCENT: Agreed.

CLINICIAN: Let's review where you are in several weeks.

To summarize, in MI, the therapist expresses empathy (through reflective listening and affirmations), develops discrepancy (between the teen's goals and behavior), avoids argumentation, rolls with resistance, and supports self-efficacy by eliciting and selectively reinforcing the client's own self-motivational statements of problem recognition, concern, desire and intention to change, and ability to change. Perhaps the most important strategy from an adolescent perspective is affirming the adolescent's freedom of choice and self-direction.

Avoiding Traps

A number of "traps" are especially relevant to working with adolescents. These traps include the (1) question–answer, (2) taking-sides, (3) expert, (4) labeling, (5) premature focus, and (6) blaming traps. In the question–answer trap, the adolescent provides only brief answers to specific, often closed-ended questions. The taking-sides trap involves the clinician advocating for a particular outcome or adolescent behavior at the expense of understanding the adolescent's ambivalence and assisting him or her in making a decision. The expert trap places the clinician in an authoritarian position relative to the adolescent, undermining any respect for adolescent autonomy. The labeling trap does exactly that; it places a diagnostic and (from an adolescent's perspective) pejorative label on the adolescent's problem rather than allowing the teen to help define it. The premature focus trap occurs when the clinician forces an intervention target before the adolescent is ready to consider that specific target. Finally, the blaming trap refers to the therapist dealing with the perceived cause of the problem rather than its solution. In MI and/or MET, adolescents are responsible for solving the problem. Emphasizing their responsibility for creating the problem only increases resistance. It is critical for the clinician to allow the adolescent to make the arguments for and against behavior change. The questions merely give the teen a framework for discussing change and perhaps resolving his or her ambivalence.

Although the fundamental processes and constituent techniques of MI are more or less used in a time sequence, each adolescent differs in his or her responses. Many of the MI techniques and skills can be used throughout most interventions. Nevertheless, MI is usually employed at the beginning of an intervention, followed by a specific modality or treatment program. An example is MI/CBT, either the 5-session version or the 12-session version, both of which have been developed for adolescents as part of the CYT trial (Dennis et al., 2004). The format of the more widely used MI/CBT 5 has two sessions of individual MI followed by three sessions of group-administered CBT. In addition to building general motivation for change, MI may also enhance motivation for engagement in CBT, or any other psychosocial intervention for adolescents with SUDs.

MI and Brief Interventions

As discussed in Chapter 1, MI is a common, if not intrinsic, part of brief interventions, which are interventions with one to four sessions, generally designed for less severe manifestations of SUDs in adolescents. For many clinicians, such as health care professionals, MI may take the form of a single session. In such venues, the clinician assists the adolescent in setting an agenda (recognizing a problem) then using such MI techniques as the readiness/importance and confidence rulers and decisional balance, and helps the adolescent resolve ambivalence and move toward preparation and intention to change. Finally, the clinician and adolescent complete a Change Plan Worksheet. Bien, Miller, and Tonigan (1993) proposed that effective brief interventions have several attributes that fit into the acronym FRAMES (feedback, responsibility, advice, menu, empathy, and self-efficacy). While I have discussed most of these components, feedback seems a bit unlike MI. Although providing feedback utilizes the clinician as expert, the clinician asks for permission to provide feedback, which is personalized information about the problem behavior and its effects presented in an objective, noncoercive way, followed by eliciting feedback from the adolescent about the feedback he or she has received. Personalized feedback consists of (1) a summary of the adolescent's substance use, especially compared with the use patterns of most adolescents within the adolescent's age group, gender, and racial or ethnic background and (2) negative consequences of the adolescent's use. For example:

> "In reviewing what you have told me about your alcohol use, your twice-weekly use until you are drunk—about 1–2 six packs—is much more frequent and a greater amount than all but a small percentage of kids your age. You have also told me that your use has affected

your relationships with your girlfriend and your parents as well as your schoolwork and attendance."

This feedback is followed by evocative questions by the clinician, such as:

"What do you make of this?"
"How does this fit or not fit with what you know about yourself?"

MI with Families and Parents

Clinicians are increasingly using MI with family members. As with individual adolescents, parents may be ambivalent about change. The flexible patient-centered, brief counseling approach of MI is congruent with the principles of family-centered care. It recognizes that the family is the expert regarding what is best for the child and assists parents to examine and resolve ambivalent feelings about health care plans and complicated medical regimens. MI includes a family-centered, supportive, and empathetic approach, with the goal of motivating parents to change or improve the teen's treatment adherence. When using the principles of MI, the first step is to develop rapport with the family. This approach requires active listening skills so that the clinician may attend to the family's fundamental beliefs regarding health and illness, including their readiness for change and confidence in making the change. Next, the clinician helps the family identify the discrepancy between desired goals and current behavior. The clinician needs to be able to roll with the family's resistance while supporting their sense of self-efficacy. The interventions involved with MI include establishing rapport, assessing behavior and motivation to change, facilitating the family's ability to make decisions and set goals, helping families with problem solving, and exchanging information. Interventions should then be tailored based on the family's readiness to change.

Potential clinical issues addressed with MI center on addictions, drug and alcohol issues, and child behavior. MI methods to be used here deal with engagement (reflection, affirming), ambivalence (reviewing pros and cons), and reduction of resistance (reflection, reframing, personal choice). As Miller and Rollnick have suggested, these strategies help keep the communication process going with patients, whether adolescents or parents. Focused use of empathy and reflective listening early in the process of working with families is designed not only to enhance the strength of the relationship but also to facilitate identifying areas of ambivalence about change. MI strategies can then be used to assess the parents' (1) desire for the situation to remain the same, (2) belief that situations can be different and that they have the ability to make the changes, (3) values and goals, and (4) competing goals and motivations (DePanfilis, 2000).

Often parents may hold a wide range of thoughts and opinions that reflect different degrees of motivation about the same topic, and thus they will be ambivalent about change. Ideal opportunities for MI arise whenever (1) clients are ambivalent about behavior changes, (2) there is evidence that the current behavior is leading to maladaptive outcomes, (3) a clear choice or choices is/are available that serve(s) the best interests of the family, and (4) an opportunity for change is realistically available. Remembering that these desires, beliefs, and motivations are fluid and can change rapidly even over the course of a single interaction is critical in the implementation of MI.

Motivational approaches can be critical for the success of treatment with adolescents with SUDs and their families. The process of asking, listening, and informing allows the clinician to help patients think about their attitudes toward change and generate their own motivations for changing behaviors. This collaborative approach, different from the more traditional, authoritative approach, enables clinicians to be catalysts for promoting behavioral change. My experience shows me time and time again that motivation can change. Adolescents and their families, when ready, will seek those who are willing to provide respect, patience, and the offer of assistance.

CONTINGENCY MANAGEMENT

Many different models of contingency management have been tried in addiction treatment settings, ranging from negative to positive reinforcement. Negative reinforcement can be seen as an extension of the parental role of "setting limits" in the form of removing privileges (e.g., access to car or computer, after-school or weekend activities) or items such as a cell phone unless expectations—compliance with treatment—are met. Any resulting motivation for treatment may not be intrinsic to the adolescent. It gets adolescents through the door of treatment, serving the same purpose as outside coercive methods such as juvenile justice or school sanctions. Just as drug courts set specific behavioral targets in terms of compliance and specify consequences of noncompliance, so too do parents need to be specific about what they are asking their teen to do with regard to compliance with assessment and/or treatment and what they will allow the adolescent to have or do as a contingency or reward. As we will discuss in Chapter 6, the parent's use of CM and rewards and consequences of adolescent behavior is a primary type of intervention used for adolescents with SUDs.

Given experience and research, positive reinforcement has been shown to be more effective than negative reinforcement and is increasingly more common. This is the case largely because this technique is therapeutic and enjoyable for both patients and staff. Negative reinforcements and punishments, though effective at times, are unpleasant to use and may result in patient dropout and other forms of resistance. Punishment, both in general and by itself, has not been a very effective method in substance abuse treatment.

CM treatments are based on a simple behavioral principle: if a behavior is reinforced or rewarded, it is more likely to occur in the future. In the case of substance abuse treatment, treatment attendance, drug abstinence, as well as other behaviors consistent with a drug-free lifestyle, can be reinforced using these principles. We can further distinguish "rewards" from reinforcers by defining "rewards" as recognition—either material or otherwise—or acknowledging that a larger goal or accomplishment has been achieved. Reinforcers are defined as smaller tokens given at a high(er) frequency for smaller, manageable behaviors or behavioral changes, thus breaking the larger goals of, say, sustained abstinence, into smaller steps such as treatment session attendance or negative drug tests.

The premise behind CM is to utilize these and other reinforcement procedures systematically to modify behaviors of substance abusers, including adolescents, in a positive and supportive manner. Contingency management can take place in two different venues: at home with parents or at a program or clinician's office; each involves different procedures. I will discuss family-based CM techniques, which we will call "contracting," in Chapter 6. (Program-based CM procedures have also been called "motivational incentives," but I will continue to refer to this as CM.)

The best example of an office- or program-based CM is the "fishbowl." The fishbowl is essentially a prize system in which attendance and drug-free urine samples are rewarded (and reinforced) with a chance to select a slip of paper from a fishbowl. Every time patients provide a drug-free (negative) urine sample, they earn a chance to draw a slip of paper from a bowl. Each draw has the possibility of winning a prize, but the patients don't always win prizes. Half of the time they draw from the bowl, they don't win anything at all: The slip says, "Good job. Keep trying" or other affirmations. About half the time, they get small prizes or gift cards (worth $1–$5). Examples include coffee shop, fast-food restaurant, or bus or public transportation cards. A few slips say "large prize" or specify a specific item; those are worth about $20 or more—like electronics or clothing—or larger gift cards. One of the slips of paper in the bowl is the jumbo prize—something like larger, more costly electronics. Variations of the fishbowl include adding another pick for each consecutive week of attendance and/or drug-free urine. For example, if the adolescent has three consecutive weeks of drug-free urines, he or she gets three selections from the fishbowl.

If they don't show up or don't have a positive urine, they get no pick, and they start over with one pick for the next attendance and/or negative urine.

It is not exactly gambling, though adolescents can get quite excited about the "chance" to win a big reward (e.g., a small TV or other electronic device). Even smaller items can be reinforcing. As attendance is often one behavioral target, the marginal increase in attendance attributable to the CM program often pays the costs of the reinforcers.

Obviously, larger reinforcers (i.e., higher value) are more potent, although intermittent reinforcement through such techniques as the fishbowl allows programs to increase the potential reward without the expense of necessarily providing it each time the target is met. If parents can afford the cost, charging them for the reinforcers seems reasonable, although some programs have found that the resulting incremental increase in attendance and revenue makes the CM program cost effective. Although CM is behaviorally based, it is theoretically neutral and can be used as an adjunct to other modalities such as MI, CBT, and family therapy or within a multimodal or 12-step-based program.

Use of CM by parents has long been a part of behavioral management of youth with disruptive behavior disorders. For adolescents with SUD, parents and adolescents develop a contract specifying both the positive and negative consequences to be delivered by parents in the event of documented abstinence or substance use. The consequences, as well as rewards, are determined via a collaborative process (see Chapter 7) between parent, adolescent, and clinician. Once formulated, the results are discussed during treatment sessions. For parental CM, other targets are possible. In keeping our operant behavioral focus, parents are taught to use liberal amounts of positive verbal reinforcement when targets or other desired behaviors are met and keep the perceived negative comments to a minimum.

SUMMARY

Increasing motivation is a critical element associated with any behavioral change, especially with adolescents and SUDs. Targeting parental motivation, MI-based intervention, and CM each represent nonexclusive methods to enhance the motivation of adolescents and their families for treatment and behavior change.

Chapter Three

The Process of Screening and Assessment

CLINICIAN: Do you drink or use drugs?
ADOLESCENT: No.
CLINICIAN: Never? Not at all?
ADOLESCENT: Well . . . sometimes, but not much.

A ssessment is the cornerstone of clinical management. Assessment often begins with screening and is usually brief or very brief, formulated to identify youth at risk for having drug or alcohol problems. Adolescents who screen positive for substance use, abuse, use disorders, or any other disorder/problem should then be given or referred for a more detailed, comprehensive assessment. Assessment defines the problem or problems. If multiple problems exist, what should the assessing clinician focus on? For adolescents, assessment at its simplest level becomes: Does the adolescent use alcohol or other illicit drugs, and what effects does this use have on the adolescent's psychosocial functioning? For screening and assessment of adolescents with substance use problems and disorders, the clinician must understand the content of assessment and should also be familiar with the process, including issues such as engagement and confidentiality.

In this chapter, I discuss the process of screening and assessment, which focuses on the context of the visit—the source and nature of the referral, confidentiality, issues relating to the validity of self-report, and engagement of the adolescent and his or her parents. The screening and assessment process involves "how to ask," and so I also review some practical techniques for interviewing adolescents and parents. The next chapter focuses on the content of screening and comprehensive assessment or "What to ask."

GATEWAYS TO SCREENING AND ASSESSMENT

What prompts a screen? For universal screening, entire populations of adolescent students are screened regardless of risk status—the likelihood that one uses substances or has an SUD. The most common reason for screening is for cause, which is either heightened risk status or the presence of specific substance use behaviors or behaviors commonly associated with substance use. Often, a parent or other adult has discovered a substance in the adolescent's possession or has found that the adolescent is intoxicated or "high." The parent or adult may be surprised at this discovery, but the more typical presentation is some level of psychosocial dysfunction as the initial concern, plus or minus a suspicion of substance use. For example, the teen is having difficulty with family relationships (e.g., arguing, being oppositional), academic functioning (getting poor grades), emotional problems (showing depression and/or anxiety), and/or has antisocial or disruptive behavior.

The range of presentations for SUDs in adolescents is almost as great as the number of adolescents with SUDs. Parents, schools, and others may refer an adolescent because of specific behaviors—for example, episodes of intoxication or an accident. More commonly, an adolescent presents with some impairment in functioning, manifested by problems at school, with peers, in family interactions, or with legal authorities. Referral sources may have some ideas about the source of the difficulties, but they seek professional guidance to confirm their suspicions or to identify the source of the problems. Intervention is all but impossible without knowing if an adolescent has a problem with substance use, the nature and severity of the problem, and what accompanying psychosocial problems are present. For example, in the case of poor academic performance, several explanations are possible, with SUDs being one possibility. Alternatively, the schoolwork could be too hard, or the teen could be depressed or anxious. Even if we establish that an adolescent has used alcohol and/or other drugs, we should not assume that any of his or her problems are necessarily the result of this use.

When an adolescent presents for screening or assessment, the reasons, venues, and timing of presentation are found to vary widely. Understanding the context of the initial visit is an important component of engaging with adolescents and their families. Often the entry point has a substantial influence on this initial contact. The clinician accepting the referral is also responsible for addressing the concerns of the referral source. When the referral is from the criminal or juvenile justice system, the concern is primarily public safety; when it comes from the family, the concerns are usually adolescent and family functioning and a general fear about the teen "getting into trouble." With referrals from school, the concern is usually academic functioning and school behavior. Other social service or mental health professionals who refer will probably have at least a modest level of knowledge about adolescents with SUDs; they will have identified you or your program as expert in assessing SUDs. While the referral source's agenda may be focused on substance use, you, as the assessing clinician, have the opportunity to assess for a broader range of problems commonly seen in adolescents with SUDs, notably serious mental health issues including suicidal or other dangerous behavior; psychosis; depressive and bipolar disorder, anxiety disorder, attention-deficit/hyperactivity disorder (ADHD), and disruptive behavior disorders (oppositional defiant disorder and conduct disorder). Because comorbidity is frequently present, the ability to identify psychopathology is sometimes as important as knowledge of substance use risks, patterns, and consequences among adolescents.

Depending on the source of referral, there might be a greater or lesser suspicion of substance use disorders. For example, a referral from most professionals, including the juvenile justice system, should indicate a higher level of suspicion of SUD owing to the likely increase in risk factors. But even those clinicians within a drug and alcohol treatment setting should resist the temptation to consider all referrals as necessarily concerned only with issues about substance use and resulting problems. Generally, referral sources are most concerned about impaired functioning from substance use, or about problems preexisting, concurrent with, or resulting from the development of SUDs, or about specific or existing general impairments in functioning. Concern about associated or concurrent problems other than SUDs is not the same as denial of substance use or SUDs. The astute clinician understands that these associated or concurrent problems may have a role in the development and maintenance of substance use or SUDs or may affect treatment response and recovery. While a narrow view of SUD treatment may look at the control of substance use behaviors as the goal for intervention, a broader and more long-term view sees improvement of psychosocial dysfunction as the goal and control of use behaviors as perhaps first among several means to that end. This is why I advise multidomain screening and assessment and attention to multiple targets, including those not obviously related to substance use. The domains to be assessed comprise the primary areas of adolescent functioning.

Professionals who refer from outside of the SUD or mental health treatment communities may not see a need to assess for substance use or related problems. However, I advise screeners to develop an index of suspicion that involves identification of high-risk teens and high-risk situations. Screening for substance use will seem obvious for those working in the fields of mental health, juvenile justice, education, and foster care, and it should be considered a routine part of assessment of youth. Referrals from primary and emergency medical care and schools, though less obvious venues, offer opportunities to screen youth with specific presentations. While youth referred from health care settings have a high index of suspicion based on their elevated number of risk factors, all professionals who work with youth should have the training and means to screen adolescents for substance use and SUDs. When appropriate levels of confidentiality are respected, parents should be informed of the professional's concerns.

School Referral

School personnel can often identify signs of trouble and refer students who need help. Schools can institute comprehensive and appropriate prevention programs and implement fair and consistent substance use policies that connect teens with needed health services. Schools, because of their access to adolescents, are in a unique position to screen them for substance use and its associated problems. Unfortunately, many view this access as an invitation to screen all students. However, screening all students may not be feasible given the prevalence of substance use among adolescents, false-positive screens for SUDs, limited access to more comprehensive assessment and treatment, and the administrative burden. The U.S. Supreme Court also forbids universal screening in the form of drug testing, but it allows schools to consider screening those involved in extracurricular activities or those receiving additional benefits (e.g., parking at school).

I advocate "for-cause" testing with sanctions only if the student does not complete recommended assessment and treatment. The ability of schools to sponsor such assessment and intervention services or use community resources to do so is varied. Student assistance programs (SAPs) provide focused services to students seeking support or needing interventions, usually for concerns related to substance use but often expanded to deal with issues of academics, attendance, behavior, mental health, or social issues. SAPs or similar policies and procedures connect programs and services within and across school and community systems to create a network of supports to help students. The SAP process identifies students in need of intervention, assesses these students' specific needs, and provides them with support and referral to appropriate resources such as treatment programs. Sources of student referrals to SAPs include school staff (e.g., school counselors), parents, or the students themselves. A SAP referral may also be part of a student's overall plan for reintegration into a school following suspension or time spent at a juvenile justice facility or in SUD treatment.

There are several different SAP models. The first, the volunteer staff model, involves existing staff (teachers, counselors, and/or other support staff) who are trained in essential SAP skills (e.g., screening, engagement, focused service), and their time is allocated to working with students and their families. The second model, the core team model, develops a program within the school and integrates SAP referral, screening, planning, and service provision. It is a variation of the volunteer/staff model described above. The core team usually consists of multidisciplinary personnel within the school (e.g., a campus administrator, school counselor, trained SAP counselor or SAP specialist, social worker, classroom teacher, school nurse, and other student services staff). A third model, the counselor model, utilizes school or community-based counseling resources to provide SAP services on a fee-for-service basis, ideally at the school. A variation of the counselor model is the community agency model involving contracts with external service providers. This latter approach, using an external agency to fully organize and administer the SAP, may be more comprehensive compared with contracting for counseling services from an individual clinician. These community providers often work with the school to establish screening and referral processes, and they make skilled clinicians available to work with students and parents. Increasingly owing to the cost of maintaining services within the school itself, school districts are utilizing the latter model of either contracting with outside providers to supply the necessary services or are maintaining lists of approved community providers from whom parents can choose to receive services. Parents are often asked to pay for these services themselves or through their health insurance. The clinician who provides SAP services or deals with school issues on behalf of their adolescent patients has additional tasks in communicating with the school and assisting their patients and parents in understanding school policies and requirements as both an advocate and liaison.

Juvenile Justice Referral

Substance use comes up as both a primary concern in the case of adolescents arrested for drug offenses (public intoxication, possession or dealing) and as an associated behavior in adolescents arrested for other violent and nonviolent offenses. Because of the high level of comorbidity of SUDs and conduct disorder and the high prevalence of SUDs in delinquent youth, almost all adolescents presenting to the juvenile justice system are at very high risk for the development or presence of SUD(s). In the case of drug offenses, the risk becomes even higher. Even with this knowledge, it is critical to systematically screen all teens entering the juvenile justice system. Screening can be administered at three points in this system: (1) at the first interview with a youth after referral to the juvenile court, often conducted by an intake officer, (2) upon admission of a youth to a pretrial detention center to await adjudication, and (3) upon admission to a postadjudication treatment or correctional program facility or provider to begin the treatment process. There are differences in the volume of cases at these three points (i.e., many more youth present at point 1), and so somewhat different screening procedures are appropriate for different points in the system. Because of the volume and relative lack of highly trained staff, screening in the juvenile justice system will often utilize screening instruments that depend less on the experience and expertise of the person screening. Ultimately, however, many of these youth will present to clinicians, who can complete more comprehensive and definitive assessments.

Perhaps the most important issue for clinicians involved with the screening of youth in the juvenile justice system is understanding their role as an agent of the court or the state. Delineating this role is especially important during preadjudication. Because of potential role conflicts and confidentiality issues, it is extremely important to maintain strict role boundaries if any treatment is initiated with detained or pretrial youths. Practical suggestions for clinicians involved in treatment include avoidance of exploration into the details or circumstances of the alleged criminal act(s), the youth's state of mind, criminal intent, mitigating factors, or defense strategies. The clinician providing court-mandated treatment may be required to submit periodic updates to the court or a designee (e.g., probation officer) regarding compliance and progress in treatment. After adjudication, the issues of any court-ordered treatments, including the clinician's role, agency, and mandated reporting to the court or probation office, should be explained to the youth and his or her family. This balancing of clinician roles and legal obligations presents a challenge to creating even a modest level of engagement with the delinquent teen. However, assuming an honest, nonconfrontational, nonjudgmental stance and advocating for the adolescent serves to promote engagement with most adolescents.

Primary Medical Care and Other Medical/Health Care Settings

Surprisingly few adolescents are identified as having problem substance use through primary care or other medical care settings. However, primary care physicians, such as pediatricians, are often the first to be asked by parents, "What should I do?" when confronted with possible substance use by their children. There are obstacles to primary care alcohol and drug-use screening, such as lack of time, training, and treatment, lack of referral resources, and unfamiliarity with available screening tools. These deficiencies have led to the development of resources to address these obstacles and to educate and train medical professionals. One example is the CRAFFT screening tool, discussed further in Chapter 4.

Primary care visits provide an opportunity for screening. The annual health maintenance visit provides a private, confidential setting in which adolescents may reasonably expect to discuss health-related behaviors and receive advice. For medical or health-related settings, specific screening tools and procedures can be administered to teens. Although a minority of referrals for the comprehensive assessment and treatment of SUDs come from health care settings, adolescents may be more receptive to both questions and advice about substance use, as they often expect health care professionals to have the teen's best interests in mind. Assurances of confidentiality, of at least the details, of substance use or other risk-taking behaviors further increase trust and the resulting accuracy of the information provided by the teenager.

Intervention for drug and alcohol problems in the hospital emergency department (ED) is consistent with the notion of a "teachable moment." There is an increased opportunity for motivation of behavior change during the critical period following a substance-related injury; patients are open to new information about their problematic substance use and are motivated to reduce their risk for substance-related injury (Newton et al., 2013). In addition to tying the accident or injury to substance use, collateral information such as that provided by biological testing can inform brief interventions as part of personalized feedback in ED settings. Often adolescents do not understand the meaning of, for example, a blood alcohol level of 0.24 mg/dl or the cognitive and motor effects of marijuana. Explaining the significance of these findings in relation to the injury they sustained can be helpful in motivating teens to modify their use of alcohol, or at least use better judgment about the circumstances under which they use alcohol or other drugs.

Parent Referral

"What are your concerns about your teen?"
"What would you like to see happen as a result of your and [adolescent's name] being here today?"

For parent-originated referrals, any level of use or problems is possible. When referred by the teen's school, juvenile justice, or primary care physicians, parents may steadfastly deny any problems or minimize their teen's behavior. Other parents may believe that their teen is experimenting and will ask for some guidance on how to handle the situation. Some parents may acknowledge that substance use is causing a significant level of conflict or psychosocial dysfunction. Finally, some parents may be convinced their child is abusing drugs despite evidence to the contrary.

Surprisingly, fewer than one in five referrals for adolescent substance abuse services comes directly from parents or the adolescents themselves. (Self-referrals by teens are particularly infrequent.) This low percentage is not necessarily due to denial that one's child is having a substance use problem; it is usually due to parental uncertainty of what to do or who to call. They may question whether there is a problem at all or whether this is merely "normal" adolescent behavior. At the very least, health care and other professionals who deal with adolescents have to be able to assist the family in answering their questions and guiding them to appropriate services.

Denial is a defense or coping mechanism. The word is often used to describe situations in which people seem unable to face reality or admit an obvious reality. Denial may be an outright refusal to admit that something has occurred, is currently occurring, or is a problem. It can also be a refusal to acknowledge the severity of a problem. Parents may display denial because the truth of the problem may hurt so much that they look for some other explanation of why their teen's behavior has changed and why he or she is experiencing problems. Both parental denial and enabling of their teen's problem are often present. In *enabling*, parents try to keep the child from experiencing the consequences of substance use (e.g., legal or school trouble) by covering up, lying for their teen, or making excuses for him or her. The stigma of having a child with substance use problems may instill a sense of shame in the parents.

Prior to formally bringing in their adolescent for a screening or assessment, parents may approach clinicians for advice on how to proceed when they suspect or know the adolescent is using substances. The clinician should first educate parents about adolescent substance use, including the developmental context, the risk factors for developing SUDs, substance use manifestations and consequences, the process of assessment, treatment planning, acute treatment, and aftercare. In many ways, the clinician's interactions with parents will mirror those with the adolescent. The clinician should be genuine and supportive; should not confront or demand; and should support self-efficacy (i.e., the parents' beliefs about their capabilities to help change their adolescent for the better). The use of MI techniques here is very useful in both engaging the parents and reducing potential resistance.

PARENT: We found a bag in Robbie's room; we think it's marijuana. My husband is not concerned as he thinks all the kids nowadays try it. But Robbie's grades have been getting worse since he started high school. Last month, he received a school suspension for talking back to a teacher. He is also more argumentative.

CLINICIAN: So, you think your son maybe using marijuana?

PARENT: I think so . . . is this normal?

CLINICIAN: While many kids try marijuana, some have problems related to its use.

PARENT: How do we know if our son has a problem or if he will develop a drug problem?

CLINICIAN: It's a problem if it gets in the way of his functioning as an adolescent—with school, with his family, and with peers. Some may get into trouble with the police. We know that some kids are more likely to develop substance use problems and disorders and continue to have those problems into adulthood if they have a family history of substance use disorders, if they have had a history of disruptive behavior when younger, and if they have mood and anxiety problems. What's important is that he is not doing well in school and has some level of impairment. Did you tell him your concerns?

PARENT: Yes, but he ignores me and goes into his room, What can we do?

CLINICIAN: We should probably arrange for an assessment. Let's discuss how you should tell him about this.

Clinicians should advise parents on what to say to their adolescent in preparation for an assessment, including how to respond to possible or expected reactions by the teen. For example, in this and future communications, clinicians should counsel parents to stay calm, regardless of how difficult that may be. Parents should also be prepared to listen to their adolescent, even if doing so is difficult owing to their adolescent's angry and perhaps abusive responses. Parents have to remain in control, as their kids are often *not* in control. In terms of the content of "the talk," parents should be specific about their concerns, especially about their worry that the teenager is or might be using alcohol or other drugs. They should avoid labels such as "druggie," "alcoholic," and "junkie" and should instead talk specifically about behaviors and negative consequences, that is, the impairments suffered by the teen and family due to substance use. Additional content suggestions for parents (adapted from *www.drugfree. org/think-child-using/your-first-step-ask*) include:

"Tell your child that you *love* him or her."
"Explain that using alcohol and other drugs can have serious consequences."
"Say it makes you *feel* worried and concerned about your child when he or she does drugs."
"Tell your child that you are there to *listen* to him or her."
"Say that you *want* him or her to be a part of the solution."
"Tell him or her what you will do to help."
"Insist that the evaluation occur."
"Don't make deals with your child."
"Do not argue with your child."

Parents are often not the primary source of the referral; rather, they bring their adolescent at the recommendation of others—the school, juvenile justice system, or primary care provider. While parents usually participate willingly in such referrals and have similar concerns as the referral source, they also have their own specific concerns and agenda. So, despite the overt reason for referral, it is always essential to ask parents—directly and specifically—what are their concerns.

The clinician should be aware of differences between the parents in their values and parenting style. Some parents may not be concerned about their teen's behavior or may label it as normative, while others may look at each teen incident of use as a violation of their norms and a cause for alarm. For example, a parent may be alarmed upon becoming aware of a single instance of substance use in the context of an otherwise highly functional adolescent. A parent's intolerance of any example of deviant behavior may be a problem. But in and of itself, the problem is not necessarily an SUD. The problem may be parent–adolescent communication, parental flexibility, and intolerance of any behaviors violating the parents' stated norms.

CONFIDENTIALITY

Adolescents are more likely to provide truthful information if they believe that their information, at least detailed information, will not be shared. Before the adolescent interview, the clinician should review exactly what information the clinician is obliged to share and with whom. Although it is obvious to the clinician that a court-ordered evaluation means a full report to the judge or probation officer, the adolescent may not be aware of this requirement. The clinician should explicitly inform the adolescent of this and similar rules. Typically, a clinician should inform the adolescent that a threat of danger to self or others makes it essential that the clinician inform a responsible adult, usually the parents, in order to keep the teenager or others safe. The clinician should also explain what he or she will have to discuss with parent(s), such as a general recommendation for treatment or impressions. The clinician should be knowledgeable about local and federal laws that limit what information may be released. Most states have confidentiality laws that restrict the information that the clinician is allowed to share with anyone unless the adolescent provides consent. This includes information about deviant behavior such as selling drugs, who sells drugs to the adolescent, and peer behaviors that include drug use and other antisocial behaviors. The clinician will have to discuss with parent(s) a general recommendation for treatment or impressions. The clinician should encourage the adolescent to reveal the extent of substance use and other problems to parents. In other cases, the clinician should discuss what information the adolescent will allow the clinician to reveal.

THE ROLE OF PARENTS IN THE ASSESSMENT PROCESS

Inclusion of parents in the screening and comprehensive assessment can be an important complement to what is done with the adolescent alone. Although parents usually only have a vague idea about the level of their adolescent's substance use, they are almost always better informants about their adolescent's overt behaviors, level of functioning, negative consequences of use, and past treatment. Since an adolescent's decision to engage and be honest is based primarily on the interviewer's candor, the adolescent must be kept informed about whether and how his parents will be included in the assessment and what they will be told. Clinicians should describe the procedure for including parents and obtain verbal confirmation that the teen understands. Parents need to be informed of the adolescent's acute status and, with the teen's encouragement and consent, be informed of precipitating or concurrent problems such as substance use, depression, and life circumstances (e.g., bullying, legal problems). All clinicians are obliged to follow rules of confidentiality. There are noted exceptions to these tenets, mentioned above, such as suspicion of physical and/or sexual abuse. However, confidentiality persists for treatment of pregnancy and sexually transmitted disease.

In most cases, however, the assessment and treatment of adolescents for substance abuse or dependence is subsumed within the types of medical treatment for which parental approval must be sought. This takes on added significance when adolescents are treated in emergency settings or where there is often a relationship between substance abuse and the need for immediate medical care. Generally, it is advisable to encourage adolescents to reveal their substance use on their own. I advise the clinician to first review with the adolescent the assessment findings, including substance use and suspicion of SUDs, before discussion with parents. Teens may be relieved if a clinician is there to assist them in informing their parents about their substance use. The best forum for discussing findings from testing and evaluation and for providing recommendations is a family meeting where everyone is available to provide input, hear the recommendations from the clinician, and verify their understanding of the plan for additional evaluation or treatment. A clinician who maintains an understanding, informative stance is more likely to produce compliance with recommendations for additional intervention than a clinician who resorts to confrontation and insistence.

ENGAGING THE PARENTS

Although parents may have arranged for assessment, the clinician should not assume a particular agenda. As previously noted, schools, the juvenile justice system, primary care providers, or other behavioral health professionals may have requested the assessment and prompted parents who may or may not feel there is a problem with substance use—or anything else for that matter. Asking about the parent's concerns is essential. For example, parents may have concerns about depression and school performance but not specifically about drug use. Regardless of the results of the assessment, the clinician must directly address the parent's presenting concerns. Three critical questions are:

"What are your concerns about [adolescent's name]?"
"What would you like to happen as a result of this meeting/evaluation/discussion?"
"How do you think I can help you?"

These questions serve to increase engagement and ultimately motivation for assessment and intervention. Often, these questions are delivered at the transition between assessment and treatment planning and/or intervention.

I generally interview the adolescent first and prior to meeting with parents, but I allow the parents time alone without the adolescent to fully express their observations and feelings. Spending time to meet with the entire family or at least parent and adolescent provides information about the interactions and communication style between parents and between parents and adolescents that is also useful for treatment planning. The clinician should try to minimize overt conflict and inflammatory negative statements about the participants. While the clinician needs to elicit the parents' opinions and reports, caution should be taken to avoid *unnecessary* negative or overly critical communications about the adolescent in the adolescent's presence. Rather than report the adolescent's history, behavior, and symptoms, the parents may angrily dismiss the adolescent as "a failure" and as "bad," or even "evil" and "out to destroy our family." I may model more appropriate ways of talking to and about each other, such as through the use of "I" statements. For example, rather than a parent saying, "You do this to drive me crazy," the parent could say, "I'm very upset about your behaviors." "Rather than say, "You're nuts!" the teen can tell his parents, "I do not think you are being fair to me." The clinician can also remind the participants to state their comments calmly and to address the person they are speaking about rather than the clinician. To prevent a parent's negative feelings about the adolescent from becoming the primary descriptors of the adolescent's behavior, the clinician should focus on specific behaviors with enough specific examples to determine a pattern of behavior rather than a short list of random events. The clinician should be proactive, demonstrating more appropriate methods of communication to family members.

Because substance use is often a covert behavior, parents often do not know the specifics of their child's use and use patterns. Optimal assessment often requires information from a variety of sources, including the adolescent, parents, other family members, school, any involved social agencies, and previous treatment records. Parents can provide important details about the adolescent's overt behavior (e.g., truancy, poor grades, aggression, opposition–defiance, secrecy) and impairments. The parent is also the preferred source of a history of early childhood behaviors and specific past interventions—both formal (through a professional) and informal (initiated by the parent without professional guidance). The parent should be able to provide information about a family history of SUDs and other psychiatric disorders, family functioning, stressors and supports, and community resources and risks.

INTERVIEWING AND ENGAGING ADOLESCENTS

The Validity of Self-Report

Substance use by adolescents is almost always a covert behavior hidden from parents, adults, and other authority figures. The clinician's and parents' knowledge of an adolescent's involvement with alcohol or other drugs may range from no knowledge or vague suspicion to awareness of significant levels of use and abuse, confirmed by both the adolescent and other informants. For any adolescent presenting with a psychosocial dysfunction or high-risk status, the clinician should develop some level of suspicion of substance use, regardless of the chief complaint or nature of the presenting problem.

In order to make evaluation and treatment decisions, clinicians need information about the teen's use and use patterns. They must obtain or try to obtain the adolescent's self-report about substance use and associated behaviors, as well as other informant reports (parents and/or siblings), and they need to synthesize information about lifestyle, behaviors, and attitudes consistent with SUDs. But can you trust what teenagers tell you? Although the clinician should always question whether any self-report about substance use is truthful, the majority of adolescents in substance abuse treatment settings or schools give temporally consistent reports of substance use.

The use of structured interviews or standardized questionnaires may also serve to support or validate the self-report. The adolescent may feel less threatened by a self-report questionnaire, either in pencil–paper form or, increasingly, in computerized forms, many of which have questions to ascertain response bias (made-up responses). The use of toxicological methods such as urine drug screens, discussed in more depth later in this book, can validate self-report by testing for the use of a specific agent. The use of urine or other toxicology has been associated with greater honesty by the adolescent.

Finally, the attitude and skill of the assessment interviewer are often the best promoters of the validity of the self-report. Engagement with the adolescent predicts more valid responses. Studies have shown that adolescents are more likely to report their own substance use accurately if they trust the clinician and feel they are being helped rather than punished.

How to Engage the Adolescent

The purpose of the screen or assessment is to obtain information. A nonjudgmental, sympathetic approach is best. Suggested tactics include seeing the adolescent first (before parents, if applicable) and beginning the interview with an initial inquiry about the adolescent's current life circumstances. This helps to reduce the level of guardedness to be expected from the adolescent. Ask about where the adolescent lives, her or his school, academic progress, home composition, relationships, friends, and preferred activities. This allows the clinician to collect information about the adolescent and his or her life and gradually engage the adolescent. The clinician should be honest with the adolescent and display genuine interest and concern about the adolescent as an independent person while withholding any display of criticism or judgment. Key aspects of the general approach are listed in Table 3.1. The following is an example:

TABLE 3.1. Approach to the Adolescent Interview

- See the adolescent first.
- Be nonjudgmental: your job is to get information.
- Ask more benign questions first—"Where he or she lives, goes to school, participates in activities?"
- Create an "index of suspicion" (from a survey of risk factors).
- Normalize behavior—"Many of the kids I take care of like to have fun with their friends. They also try alcohol. What about you?"
- "How much do you drink or use?"

"Sarah, tell me where you live."
"What's it like living there?"
"Whom do you live with? Any brothers or sisters? Do you get along? With your folks?"
"Where do you go to school? What's it like there?"
"Tell me about your friends. Tell me about your best friends. What are they like? What do you like to do with them?"
"Are you satisfied with your friends? Do you think you have enough friends?"

In identifying the adolescent's behavioral patterns and environmental milieu, the clinician surveys the number and types of risk factors present and can then determine whether the adolescent fits a high-risk profile. If an adolescent indeed fits such a profile and there are corroborating reports of use from parents or the school, the clinician may be less dependent on the adolescent's self-report to reach a reasonable level of suspicion that the adolescent is abusing alcohol and/or other drugs. For example, an adolescent over the age of 13 with the presence of childhood-onset ADHD, oppositional–defiant behaviors, poor anger control, aggression, family history of parental SUDs, and current family and school difficulties is at very high risk for substance use and SUDs and should have a careful assessment of substance use patterns. The presence of multiple risk factors demand a careful, comprehensive assessment, which forms the basis of treatment planning and intervention.

As with any clinical interview with youth, you must identify the adolescent's developmental and cognitive level in order to ask questions in an appropriate manner and understand the adolescent's answers. Adolescents who abuse substances have a high frequency of developmental and learning disabilities and delays. An individual adolescent's facility with expressive and receptive language may lag considerably behind his or her chronological age.

Asking about Substance Use

Generally, few clinicians outside of those regularly treating adolescents with SUDs are comfortable asking or answering questions about substance use. If the clinician is uncomfortable, the adolescent may sense this feeling and increase his or her own apprehension about the interview. Hopefully, the initially benign line of questioning settles everyone down and engages the adolescent. Going from asking about peers and activities with peers to asking about parties and substance use is often a good strategy. "Partying" is often a euphemism for an alcohol and/or other drug-use episode. In a matter-of-fact manner, ask if the teen goes to parties with friends or just "hangs out"; then ask about substance use. Initially, one can ask an open question: "Tell me about your alcohol (drug) use." For those high on an index of suspicion, I ask how frequently they use (particularly alcohol and marijuana), assuming a positive response. Be prepared for vague answers such as "a little," "sometimes," "not much," or even "a lot." But do not be satisfied with these responses: demand a clear answer—even an estimate for most weeks in terms of frequency and quantity. Offer options—daily, almost every day, two to three times per week—and allow the teen to respond. Quantity is often difficult to ascertain for many drugs, except alcohol. For alcohol, interestingly, individual drinks or servings of beer, wine, or spirits have approximately the same amount of alcohol. So one can ask how many drinks over an episode of drinking without necessarily distinguishing between types of alcohol.

CLINICIAN: How often do you use marijuana?

ADOLESCENT: Not much.

CLINICIAN: How many times a week? Once a week, two to three times, or every day—or almost every day?

ADOLESCENT: Weekends usually.

CLINICIAN: Both Saturday and Sunday?

ADOLESCENT: Yes, usually.

CLINICIAN: Ever on school days? Other days during the week?

ADOLESCENT: Maybe one to two more days, occasionally almost every day.

CLINICIAN: How many times each day?

ADOLESCENT: Once or twice.

CLINICIAN: Ever more?

ADOLESCENT: Sometimes on Saturday . . . all day.

Adolescents may also be willing to share information about anonymous friends, including the friends' alcohol and drug use. If the adolescent reports numerous friends using and/or abusing alcohol and other drugs, attending parties where use is present, and if the adolescent fits into other "high-risk" characteristics, the clinician's suspicion of substance use should be raised even further.

The purpose of an initial visit for assessment is to obtain as much information as possible; therefore, the clinician should avoid any unnecessary confrontation that may compromise accurate, reliable reporting. Inconsistencies should initially be probed gently. For example, when an adolescent states that she has tried beer only twice, both times at friends' parties, the clinician may ask, "I'm a little confused. You told me before that you never went to a party where there was alcohol or other drugs." Later, when the clinician provides the adolescent and his or her family with feedback, a more pointed, direct approach is often both necessary and effective. As the "expert," you will have to provide your professional opinion, whether the adolescent likes it or not. Honesty in the context of offering help—for both the parents' and adolescent's agendas—may soften the "bad news" for the adolescent and make your summary and subsequent recommendations more palatable.

When a more substantial history of alcohol or other drug use is suspected, the clinician should calmly state the suspicions and offer help and understanding if the adolescent chooses to be honest with the interviewer. The interviewer should give the teen several opportunities to set the record straight about his or her substance use, including level of use. Frequent summaries of previous answers allow the adolescent to "correct" the interviewer.

> "Sarah, let me see if I understand what you are telling me. . . . You started drinking when you were 13 years of age and over the last several months, you usually drank until you had a buzz on, on weekends—that's two times a week? You get really drunk maybe once a month."

Summarizing consequences is also useful, but direct confrontation is generally not advised. An adolescent rarely responds positively to being told, "I don't believe you," or "I think that you're lying." The increase in resistance translates to the teen not cooperating or providing information. At the same time, expressions of appreciation for the teen's honesty and effort may increase valid reports. Affirmations (see Chapter 2) may also increase engagement and the teen's perception that the clinician is there to help.

"Sometimes it can be difficult to admit this to an adult, especially your parents." Or "I appreciate your being honest with me. That can't be easy. It must be important for you to give me an honest report."

During the screening interview, open-ended questions and reflective listening increase the adolescent's engagement and promote discussion about the perceived negative consequences of drug use. This is an important strategy in motivational interviewing and an important first step toward intervention. Ultimately, these strategies may lead to greater receptivity to behavior changes. During the interview, the clinician can assess the adolescent's current attitude toward change, which may be helpful in guiding further intervention. Prochaska and DiClemente (1983), in their transtheoretical model, conceptualized change as a process involving progress through a series of stages (see Table 3.2). During the course of an assessment interview, the clinician will have opportunities to ascertain the level of the adolescent's motivation and stage of change. Often, these inquiries should take the form of direct questions.

"Given the problems that you and your parents have reported as a result of your drug use, have you considered stopping or decreasing use? Have you taken any steps toward changing? What keeps you from changing?"

TABLE 3.2. Stages of Change

1. *Precontemplation:* No change is being considered, as the adolescent is either unaware that his or her behavior is problematic or has never considered change.

2. *Contemplation:* The adolescent is beginning to recognize that his or her substance use is problematic and starts to consider change, including the "pros and cons" of change versus continued use.

3. *Preparation:* The adolescent expresses the intent to take action toward reducing or stopping substance use in the immediate future and may begin taking small steps toward change.

4. *Action:* The adolescent has taken specific actions toward making positive change in his or her substance use.

5. *Maintenance:* The adolescent has made change and wishes to continue.

6. *Termination:* The adolescent expresses no desire to use and is certain of his or her ability to control use.

Note. Adapted from Prochaska and DiClemente (1983).

Clinicians do not always express their concern and caring explicitly to their adolescent patients, but expressing caring and empathy, as well as promoting a patient's self-efficacy, are useful strategies for prompting both engagement and behavioral changes. Such messages might take the form of "I am very worried about you" or "That sounds like a lot [of substance use]." These sentiments may prepare adolescents who are high-risk substance users to accept the next step toward treatment.

DRUG TESTING

Toxicological tests of bodily fluids (usually urine but also saliva, blood, and hair samples) to detect the presence of specific substances should be part of the formal evaluation and the ongoing assessment of substance use. The optimal use of urine screening requires proper collection techniques, including the monitoring of obtaining the sample, evaluation of positive results, and specific plan(s) of action should the specimen be positive or negative for the presence of substance(s). Prior to testing, the clinician should establish rules regarding the confidentiality of the results. Because of the limited time a drug will remain in the urine, as well as possible adulteration of the sample, a negative urine test does not indicate that the adolescent does not use drugs. A positive specimen indicates only the presence of specific drug(s) and not necessarily the presence of an SUD or a specific pattern of use.

Drug testing is often part of SUD treatment programs. Inexpensive urine drug test kits are readily available for use in programs and even at home. These are qualitative tests in that they measure the presence (or absence) of a specific substance or panel of substances in the urine at concentrations above a specific threshold. To track changes in substance concentration in the urine over time, especially with tetrahydrocannabinol (THC), the primary psychoactive ingredient in marijuana, one requires the use of quantitative drug tests, which are more costly.

If drug testing has not been legally mandated, clinicians cannot realistically force an adolescent to undergo it. The clinician should inform both parents and the adolescent that the clinician may request drug testing at any time and that a refusal to submit to testing will be considered a "positive" result. The clinician should also tell parents that he or she cannot reveal test results unless the adolescent provides permission. (This is usually in the form of a signed release of information.) However, clinicians should allow, and even encourage, parents to use negative (e.g., threat of punishment, restriction) or positive (rewards) reinforcement so that the teen allows communication about drug testing results. The important aspect of drug testing is that a plan needs to be developed with both adolescents and parent(s). Such a plan must include the stipulation that a urine sample will be provided by the adolescent upon request of either parent or treatment professional, and it should specify contingencies that depend on whether the sample is positive or negative. I advise parents to use home drug testing kits only under the supervision of a professional and as part of a comprehensive treatment plan. On their own, parents usually have not considered the consequences or contingencies of home drug testing. Positive results portend a crisis when a frantic parent calls his or her pediatrician, family doctor, or other professional, asking "What do we do now?!" What happens with a positive result, or even a negative result, should be determined before drug testing begins.

The specific procedures for obtaining urine samples include:

- Provision of a sample upon request, which may be random or scheduled (weekly or biweekly).
- No coats, loose clothing, or fluids allowed into the restroom.
- The sample handed directly to the clinician or to a representative of the treatment program.

The sample should be warm (close to body temperature) and not appear overly diluted. Many drug testing kits have an indicator of temperature, and some indicate specific gravity to identify samples that are overly dilute. Water is the most common adulterant, so a dilute sample may represent an effort to get a negative result, as the dilution lowers the concentration of the substance in the sample. In my experience, kits with such measures considerably lower the risk of adulteration. Entirely eliminating the risk requires direct visualization of the sample entering the container. Direct visualization is highly intrusive and often requires clinicians of both genders. Visualization should be reserved for adolescents who have provided or been suspected of providing adulterated urine samples. Guidelines for drug testing are summarized in Table 3.3.

Because adolescents often present to me acknowledging broad, often significant, levels (quantity and frequency) of specific substance use, I may not use drug testing at initial evaluation since it would be redundant. However, I consider drug testing an essential part of treatment and ongoing follow-up. When I do utilize urine drug tests to validate the negative use report of an adolescent strongly suspected or at very high risk for substance use, I explain to teens and parents alike that this is done routinely as a validity check on adolescent reports. Regardless of adolescents' frequent protest of privacy invasion or lack of trust, I will obtain a sample or consider a refusal to provide the sample as a positive result.

TABLE 3.3. Guidelines for Urine Drug Testing/Screening

- Explain the rationale and procedures to the adolescent and parent(s).

- Most state laws support the contention that the adolescent has a right to refuse testing and, if tested, to keep results private unless he or she gives the clinician permission to disclose results to parents.

- Parents and the clinician should attempt to obtain permission for release of testing results.

- Assuming consent, the adolescent should always be prepared to give a sample.
  □ Refusal to submit a sample equals a positive result.
  □ Sampling can be random.

- Determine in advance what happens if the test is positive or negative.

- Witness collection of samples for adolescents suspected of adulterating them.
  □ Make direct observation.
  □ Prevent substitution, dilution, and adulterants.

- A positive test does not necessarily indicate a problem or SUD diagnosis.

SUMMARY

The validity and reliability of both screening and comprehensive assessment require engagement and communication with the adolescent and his or her parent(s) in hopes of building trust and obtaining information essential for treatment planning. The clinician should consider the source of the referral and the context of the assessment, including involvement in various systems such as medical, juvenile justice, school, and child welfare. Important considerations are keeping and explaining confidentiality and the use of drug screens as an adjunct to self-reports.

Chapter Four

The Content of Screening and Assessment

I n this chapter, I focus on the content of screening and assessment—what to ask. It includes domains of adolescent functioning: substance use and its associated behaviors; emotional and behavioral symptoms; school, family, and peer functioning; and medical problems. Finally, I consider the use of assessment instruments.

SCREENING

An optimal screen is a brief series of questions that seek information on the elements of both substance use and dysfunction. Screens are not the final word in determining the nature of the problem or whether an SUD actually exists. Rather, screening is a method of decreasing the number of adolescents requiring a more detailed time- and cost-intensive comprehensive assessment.

Some adolescents, by virtue of their legal status (delinquent) or involvement in one or more other systems of care, may require routine universal screening. I strongly recommend routine screening of all youth in the juvenile justice or foster care systems or those with mental health problems. There is a high prevalence of SUDs in those populations, and most will require a more comprehensive assessment. For most health and behavioral care professionals and for educators, screening is done on a "for-cause" basis due to the presence of (1) health problems that might be substance related, such as accidents or injury, changes in eating or sleeping patterns, the presence of sexually transmitted diseases, chronic pain, or pregnancy; or (2) substantial behavioral changes, such as increased oppositional–defiant behavior, change of friends or peer group, deterioration in grades, significant mood changes, repeated unexcused school absences, or loss of interest in previously preferred activities.

Simple Brief Screens

Although screening is meant to be brief, some screens are briefer than others. Simple screens should not include more than a few (six or fewer) questions. Comprehensive screens are longer and usually include screening questions for other problems. Screens can be delivered verbally and via a paper-and-pencil or computer-based instrument.

As discussed in Chapter 3, in a verbal screen, the screener should start the conversation with less threatening or less emotionally charged topics such as school, friends, and the teen's perception of home life. Because of the importance of primary care screening of adolescents for substance use, the American Academy of Pediatrics (AAP) has provided clinical guidance on the use of a system for screening and intervention with adolescents seen in primary care settings. That system consists of screening, brief intervention, and referral to treatment (SBIRT) and can also be used in other medical settings (e.g., emergency departments, health clinics). SBIRT is backed by a solid research base for adults, although the research support for SBIRT for adolescents is much less established (Levy, Williams, & the Committee on Substance Use and Prevention, 2016; AAP, 2011). Over the past decade, adolescent models of SBIRT have been developed. One principle underlying SBIRT is that screening may reveal varying levels of substance use involvement, ranging from abstinence to dependence, and should result in commensurate interventions ranging from advice or brief intervention to specific SUD treatment.

For alcohol-only screening, a brief verbal screen recommended by the National Institute on Alcohol Abuse and Alcoholism (NIAAA; 2007) can be used by busy pediatricians or other primary medical professionals. It asks two key questions to screen about alcohol use in adolescents.

For children ages 9–11 and adolescents 11–14, the health care professional asks:

> "Do you have any friends who drank beer, wine, or any drink containing alcohol in the *past year*?"

Followed by:

"In the *past year, on how many days* have you had more than a few sips of beer, wine, or any drink containing alcohol?"

For older adolescents, ages 14–18, the questions are asked in the reverse order—about the adolescent first, then:

"If your friends drink, *how many drinks* do they usually drink on an occasion?"

For youth less than 14 years of age, any drinking is cause for concern. Figure 4.1 shows who is at highest risk and at moderate risk for having alcohol problems by age. Level of risk helps determine the level of intervention (see Chapter 5). A pattern or multiple episodes of binge drinking (defined as three to five or more drinks per occasion) also prompts increased concern about problem drinking. Screening questions for alcohol can be reduced even further to one key question about the frequency of alcohol use with specific thresholds. For early and middle adolescents (ages 12–14 and 15–17, respectively), a report of ≥3 days in the past year, and for older adolescents (those 17 or older) ≥12 drinking days per year, should prompt more detailed assessment (Clark et al., 2016).

For screening for both alcohol and other drugs of abuse, the AAP (Levy et al., 2016) presents three other instruments, the CRAFFT, the

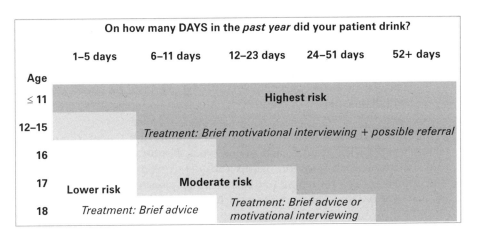

FIGURE 4.1. Alcohol screening paradigm: Estimated risk levels by age and frequency in the past year. From National Institute on Alcohol Abuse and Alcoholism (2014).

Brief Screener for Tobacco, Alcohol and other Drugs (BSTAD), and the Screening to Brief Intervention (S2BI) tool.

CRAFFT is an acronym, with each letter standing for a key word in the seven questions constituting the screen (see Figure 4.2). The CRAFFT, usually administered in interview form, is a six-item screen developed by Knight and his colleagues (2002) and consists of unambiguous questions that can cover alcohol as well as other substances (Knight et al., 2002). The AAP originally recommended the CRAFFT for use with adolescents because of the tool's simplicity, practicality, and psychometrics. Allowing for a quick screen of any substance use behavior, the CRAFFT quickly screens simultaneously for alcohol and other drug use disorders (AAP, 2011).

The CRAFFT screen consists of two parts: the first question should be asked of all adolescents, and the following should only be asked of those who answered "yes" to any of the opening questions regarding personal substance use: "Have you ever drunk alcohol?"; "Have you ever smoked marijuana?"; "Have you ever used another substance to get high?" Each "yes" response on CRAFFT is 1 point. A score of 2 or greater is a positive screen and indicates that the adolescent is at higher risk for having an alcohol- or drug-related disorder. Lower scores (2–4) indicate a need for brief advice or brief interventions, while higher scores suggest not only brief advice/intervention but also referral for intensive treatment. The CRAFFT is reasonably sensitive, specific, and predictive, and the established validity is not significantly affected by age, gender, or race/ethnicity.

"Have you ever drunk alcohol?"
"Have you ever smoked marijuana?"
"Have you ever used another substance to get high, including illicit drugs, over-the-counter preparations, prescription medications, inhalants, herbs, or plants?"

If a teen has endorsed the use of two or more substances, the clinician should review use of each major type of substance. To maximize the sensitivity, each question begins with "Have you ever . . . ?" unless the adolescent is a returning patient, in which case the questions begin, "Since your last appointment/visit/session. . . ." For those teens who have already informed you of use or who are aware that you know of their use (e.g., parents have told you in their presence), the clinician can proceed directly to screen quantity, frequency, and consequences. Adolescents whose high-risk status is known may be presumed to use; queries such as "How often?" or "How much do you use" may result in a more honest acknowledgment of use.

To be completed by the patient

Please answer all questions **honestly**; your answers will be kept **confidential**.*

During the PAST 12 MONTHS, on how many days did you:

1. Drink more than a few sips of beer, wine, or any drink containing **alcohol**? Put "0" if none.

    # of days

2. Use any **marijuana** (pot, weed, hash, or in foods) or **"synthetic marijuana"** (like "K2" or "Spice")? Put "0" if none.

    # of days

3. Use **anything else to get high** (like other illegal drugs, prescription or over-the-counter medications, and things that you sniff or "huff")? Put "0" if none.

    # of days

READ THESE INSTRUCTIONS BEFORE CONTINUING:

If you put "0" in ALL of the boxes above, ANSWER QUESTION 4, THEN STOP.

If you put "1" or higher in ANY of the boxes above, ANSWER QUESTIONS 4–9.

	No	Yes
4. Have you ever ridden in a **CAR** driven by someone (including yourself) who was "high" or had been using alcohol or drugs?	☐	☐
5. Do you ever use alcohol or drugs to **RELAX**, feel better about yourself, or fit in?	☐	☐
6. Do you ever use alcohol or drugs while you are by yourself, or **ALONE**?	☐	☐
7. Do you ever **FORGET** things you did while using alcohol or drugs?	☐	☐
8. Do your **FAMILY** or **FRIENDS** ever tell you that you should cut down on your drinking or drug use?	☐	☐
9. Have you ever gotten into **TROUBLE** while you were using alcohol or drugs?	☐	☐

*Two or more YES answers suggest a serious problem and need for further assessment.

FIGURE 4.2. CRAFFT Questionnaire (version 2.0). Copyright © John R. Knight, MD, Boston Children's Hospital. Reproduced by permission from the Center for Adolescent Substance Abuse Research (CeASAR), Boston Children's Hospital. For more information and versions in other languages, see *www.ceasar.org*.

CLINICIAN: Tell me about some of the activities that you do with your friends.

ADOLESCENT: I mess around—play video games, skateboard.

CLINICIAN: Do you ever "party" with your friends?

ADOLESCENT: Huh?

CLINICIAN: You know, have a good time, after you skateboard. Do you drink—beer, wine, or the hard stuff, smoke marijuana?

ADOLESCENT: Eh . . . yeah, sometimes beer.

CLINICIAN: When you drink—how often, how many times a week or month?

ADOLESCENT: Not much.

CLINICIAN: But how often, on average, in the average week?

ADOLESCENT: Just on weekends.

CLINICIAN: How often do you get drunk?

ADOLESCENT: Probably at least one time a week—the other times I just get a buzz on.

CLINICIAN: How much do you drink each time? How many drinks?

ADOLESCENT: Usually a friend and I share a six-pack. His brother keeps cases in the fridge in their garage.

CLINICIAN: Has anything bad ever happened when you were drinking? Has anyone (adult) caught you? Have you ever gotten in trouble?

ADOLESCENT: Yeah, my folks caught me last week—I think that's why I am here.

CLINICIAN: What about marijuana?

If any of the opening questions is answered "yes," the clinician should administer a formal screen, developmentally appropriate and validated for use with adolescents. These are discussed later in this chapter.

The following dialogue is another example of how to screen substances and frequency of use.

CLINICIAN: Many of the kids I take care of like to have fun with their friends. They also try alcohol. What about you?

ADOLESCENT: Eh . . . yeah, I tried it. I've drunk alcohol before.

CLINICIAN: Have you been drunk before?

ADOLESCENT: Yeah.

CLINICIAN: In the last 3 months, how often do you drink?

ADOLESCENT: Not much, sometimes.

CLINICIAN: How much is that? Once a week, several times a week, once or several times a month?

ADOLESCENT: I guess several times a month.

CLINICIAN: How often do you get drunk? Most of these times?

ADOLESCENT: Most but not every time. Mostly to get a buzz.

CLINICIAN: What about marijuana? Other drugs—like pills not prescribed to you, cocaine, or LSD?

ADOLESCENT: Maybe once a month—but I don't use anything else.

CLINICIAN: I appreciate your sharing this information with me. Do you have any concerns about using alcohol or other drugs? How about friends or family—are they ever concerned?

Simple screens based on frequency of use have their limitations. One can expect a significant number of adolescents to report at least some use of substances. For example, an overwhelming majority of teens will report some exposure to alcohol, and a significant minority have some experience with marijuana. Small amounts or infrequent use will probably identify a large population of adolescents to whom administering a more comprehensive assessment would be impractical. Screening should inquire about dysfunction and/or distress associated with levels of substance use. Most screens are based on the following "use plus" concept. First, the adolescent has to have a pattern of use. One to two episodes of use of a specific substance would not meet this threshold unless there were severe consequences. Once a threshold for frequency is met, a screen will also include a brief survey of direct consequences of use or salient drug use behaviors. The CRAFFT may be limited by its reliance on "yes" responses to indicate the true extent of substance use–related problems. Regardless of its limitations, the CRAFFT begins a conversation between the adolescent and a health care professional.

Similarities exist between the CRAFFT and two more recently developed instruments designed for primary settings. The BSTAD uses highly sensitive and specific cutoffs to identify various SUDs among adolescents 12–17 years of age: ≥ 6 days of past-year use for tobacco and >1 day of past-year use for alcohol or marijuana (Kelly et al., 2014). The S2BI (see Figure 4.3) instrument can be administered digitally and uses a stem question and forced-response options (none, once or twice, monthly, and weekly or more) in a sequence to indicate the frequency of past-year use of tobacco, alcohol, marijuana, and five other classes of substances most commonly used by adolescents (Levy, Siqueira, & the Committee on Substance Abuse, American Academy of Pediatrics, 2014; Levy et al., 2016). The

Introduction: I'm going to ask you a few questions that I ask all my patients; please be honest. I will keep your answers confidential.

In the past year, how many times have you used:

	Never	Once or twice	Monthly	Weekly
• Tobacco?				
• Alcohol?				
• Marijuana?				

STOP if all "Never." Otherwise, CONTINUE.

	Never	Once or twice	Monthly	Weekly
• Prescription drugs that were not prescribed for you (such as pain medication or Adderall)?				
• Illegal drugs (such as cocaine or Ecstasy)?				
• Inhalants (such as nitrous oxide)?				
• Herbs or synthetic drugs (such as salvia, "K2," or bath salts)?				

S2BI Results and Scoring: Administer the first three questions. Stop if all "Never." Otherwise, administer next set of questions and follow the instructions below based on the received responses.

No Use—Provide positive reinforcement of current behaviors.

Couple of Times—Deliver second set of questions • Provide brief advice.

Monthly Use—Deliver second set of questions • Assess further using CRAFFT tool • Perform recommended action based on CRAFFT score.

Weekly Use—Deliver second set of questions • Assess further using CRAFFT tool • Perform recommended action based on CRAFFT score.

FIGURE 4.3. S2BI: Screening to Brief Intervention. Copyright © 2014 Boston Children's Hospital. All rights reserved. This work is licensed under a Creative Commons Attribution—NonCommercial 4.0 International License.

S2BI is highly sensitive and specific in discriminating among clinically relevant use-risk categories, allowing it to more directly detect possible DSM-5 SUDs, as the adolescent's response to questions about frequency of substance use in the past year correlates to the likelihood of having a SUD. For example, answers of "monthly use" suggest mild or moderate SUD, while answers of "weekly or more" correlate with a severe SUD.

Accident-related behaviors are common in adolescents and include taking chances on bicycles or skateboards, not using seat belts, driving over the speed limit, or riding with reckless or even intoxicated drivers. Substance use compounds these risks, and a surprising number of adolescents acknowledge these activities while under the influence. In venues such as the emergency department (ED), the appearance of adolescents with injuries should immediately arouse suspicion of acute substance use or intoxication. Other characteristics, especially those associated with increased risk for substance use and SUDs (e.g., ADHD, depression, association with deviant peers), may further increase suspicion. Clinicians should critically examine all accidents and not just those involving motor vehicles. The adolescent's concern about his or her own health may be enough to prompt cooperation and a truthful report. Establishing rapport with the adolescent, even in this stressful setting, is critical to the screening process. MI techniques are useful. A clinician might start by inquiring about the adolescent's view of what happened and why there is a need for emergency care. The items from the CRAFFT can be interspersed in the discussion of the adolescent's view of his or her need for treatment. This allows the screen not only for SUDs but also for other high-risk behaviors such as unprotected sex. Tying the adolescent's substance use to his or her current circumstances can occasionally produce some insight and desire to change. Ultimately, a clinical judgment can be made about whether adolescents are engaging in behaviors that place them at risk for future injury and whether they should be referred for additional evaluation and treatment.

If the adolescent does not use substances and endorses only occasional or sporadic use of alcohol or marijuana without any impairment or other risk-taking behaviors, the clinician should reinforce the adolescent's choice of abstinence and advise that health is better served by avoiding substance use.

> "It looks like you have made some good choices in not using marijuana or other drugs. We know that kids who do use have more problems—such as health, school, and home issues—than those, like you, who don't use. Do you think there will be any obstacles in the future that might keep you from being abstinent—that is, not using? Peer pressure? Difficulty saying no to your friends?"

Or

"I know that your alcohol use now does not sound like much, but it's easy to slip into bad habits. Do you think you might use more or try more substances in the future? What might encourage you to use? And what might keep you from using?"

For adolescents who endorse more substance use, including regular patterns of use and minor problems or impairments, brief interventions (covered in Chapter 5) offer a potentially effective intervention short of referral for specific SUD treatment.

Standardized Screening Instruments

In contrast to simple screens, a number of screening instruments are available that tap into multiple domains of functioning (see Table 4.1). Both clinicians and nonclinicians use screening instruments to identify adolescents at risk for substance abuse, those already with substance abuse, and those meeting a minimum threshold of problematic behavior who require more detailed assessment to determine their substance use status. The use of normed, standardized instruments for screening allows individuals with a very modest level of training to complete or supervise completion of the screening. The use of screening interviews such as the Teen Addiction Severity Index (T-ASI; Kaminer, Wagner, Plumer, & Seifer, 1993) does require training and experience. There are two types of screening instruments: unidomain and multidomain. Unidomain instruments measure a specific area, most likely substance use and directly related behaviors. Examples of unidomain instruments include the Adolescent Alcohol Involvement Scale (AAIS; Mayer & Filstead, 1979), Adolescent Drinking Index (ADI; Harrell & Wirtz, 1989), Rutgers Alcohol Problem Index (RAPI; White & Labouvie, 1989), and Alcohol Use Disorders Identification Test (AUDIT; Knight, Sherritt, Harris, Gates, & Chang, 2003). Multidomain instruments assess a wider range of variables including behaviors, psychiatric symptoms, family and school functioning, and attitudes. Multidomain instruments are likely to be more useful to clinicians and researchers. In addition to information about substance use, multidomain instruments assess other areas of adolescent functioning that may be affected by the substance use. Examples of multidomain screening instruments include the Drug Use Screening Inventory (DUSI; Tarter, 1990) and Problem Oriented Screening Instrument for Teenagers (POSIT; Santisteban, Tajeda, Dominicis, & Szapocznik, 1999), which are available in both paper-and-pencil and computer formats.

Screening Feedback

Providing feedback on the results of the screen to both the teen and his or her parents is essential. Adolescents should be given a nonjudgmental summary of the facts—that their use is above what most teens use, that they are at risk for suffering consequences from use—in both the short and the long term—according to the research. There should be no moralizing, no shaming or labeling! (See Table 3.1 for how to approach the adolescent.)

If the adolescent denies substance use or is below the threshold for concern, the clinician should praise his or her choices of not using and of having nonusing friends. The clinician may wish to elicit and affirm reasons to not use substances: "So, what made you decide not to drink [or use] . . . ?" If friends use, then the clinician may add, " . . . especially when your friends use?" If the teen appears open to input, you may want to help him or her to understand the consequences of substance use on brain development and that use at an early age increases the risk for serious alcohol problems later in life. Even sporadic use or intoxication can lead to impaired sensory–motor functioning (e.g., driving, biking, skateboarding, and swimming can lead to accidents) and faulty judgment. Finally, explore how the teen plans to stay alcohol free when friends use, asking for their ideas on handling situations where they may feel pressure to use. Always advise against riding in a car with a driver who has been drinking or using other drugs, especially if they are that driver.

> "Sounds like you have tried marijuana but did not like the way it made you feel (or decided that it was not worth getting into trouble or something bad happening), so you did not use again. A lot of teenagers feel that way too. Many adolescents do develop more serious problems, particularly if they start to use marijuana regularly—or even every day. As a medical professional, I see a lot of accidents—not just in cars but involving bicycles and skateboards—involving marijuana or other drug or alcohol use. I give you a lot of credit. It is not easy to avoid using. I know there is a lot of peer pressure to use. Is that the case for you? My experience in talking with adolescents is that kids do better when they think about decisions like using or being pressured to use beforehand so that they can figure out a way to respond in a way they feel more comfortable with."

For adolescents who endorse use, particularly above the screening threshold, the clinician may ask if teens feel their use is a problem. The clinician should further explain that the adolescent scored above the threshold, that the clinician is concerned and is recommending that the adolescent receive more comprehensive assessment.

CLINICIAN: I administered a screening scale to you, and it indicated that you were at increased risk of having problems with drugs/or alcohol. What do you make of that?

ADOLESCENT: Well, I don't know, Doc. I don't think I have a problem.

CLINICIAN: And you may not . . . but I am here to help you stay healthy, so I need to let you know when I see risks to your health. I know from research that even kids who only occasionally use drugs or alcohol may have more difficulty driving or even skateboarding and have many more accidents than teens who do not use. Because your brain has not quite reached your final adult level, drugs and alcohol use may affect brain development. That may limit how well you do in high school, college, or technical school and how good a job you eventually get. Also, the earlier someone starts using, the more likely they will eventually develop problems with their use, including consequences such as affecting schoolwork and relations with your family and some of your friends. So what do you think? What would you like to do?

ADOLESCENT: Well, I guess I need to think about it. But you cannot make me stop!

CLINICIAN: Yes, you are correct. No one can *make* you stop. You may have some consequences from your use, but the decision to use—or not to use—is up to you.

ADOLESCENT: I am not sure I am ready to stop, maybe later. . . .

CLINICIAN: Sometimes, kids find making a little experiment useful—a trial period off from using drugs or alcohol—say for 1–2 months. Maybe this is something that you could try. We can see what happens to your grades, how well you get along with your parents. Then you can decide whether continuing your use works for you and whether to use or not after that.

According to the SBIRT model, positive screens will often lead to brief intervention.

Those who utilize screening procedures for substance use and SUDs should also be acquainted, if not skilled, in such brief interventions, which can serve as stand-alone interventions as well as bridges to more substantial interventions for substance use problems.

ADOLESCENT: I don't know. I think my friends would give me a hard time if I don't use.

CLINICIAN: I can imagine that would be tough. But thinking about what you might say ahead of time is helpful. You could come up with a plan. What could you say?

ADOLESCENT: I could say I don't feel like it today or . . . I have to do my homework or babysit later.

CLINICIAN: Those are all good ideas! Let me know if you need additional help. I know folks who really know about these types of issues and work well with teenagers like you.

ADOLESCENT: I don't want to go to rehab!

CLINICIAN: No, this is someone who you can talk with as an outpatient. Whatever you decide to do after that is your own and your parents' choice.

Alternatively, the clinician could say:

"I would really like you to visit with some folks who know about these kinds of issues and would help you determine just what extra help you may—or may not—need."

Owing to confidentiality issues, the clinician may not be able to detail the specifics of the adolescent's substance use to the parents. Generally, expressing concern about the teen's behavior and advising the family about the need for a more comprehensive assessment is sufficient. Attempting to align with the teen and supporting him or her in their disclosure to parents is also a useful technique in lieu of having to reveal the details of the adolescent's behavior.

CLINICIAN: As part of your son's regular physical exam, we administered some screens to try to pick up any problems before they get worse or early enough to make interventions easier. I know that you have mentioned some concern that he may be smoking and drinking.

PARENT: Yes, we caught him at his brother's house, drinking beer with his friends.

CLINICIAN: Well, he has given me permission to let you know that his screen for alcohol was positive, meaning that he drinks more than most kids his age and that he may have problems.

PARENT: Is he an alcoholic?

CLINICIAN: No, but his use may be affecting his school progress and other aspects of his functioning. Clearly, however, we need more information about his substance use and perhaps other problems that teenagers often experience. If it is all right with you, I can give you the names of professionals who can do this and help your son.

Alternatively, the clinician could say:

"Although your son may drink more than most of his peers, the frequency is not high, and he appears to be functioning fairly well. He appears to understand that his alcohol use has some risks. I think we can watch and monitor his alcohol use and overall functioning. As parents, it is important that you monitor his activities—where he is at and where he is going, who he is with, and when he is coming home. I am going to provide you with some information that may help you do this. If anything changes or you have questions, please let me know."

Knowledge of providers and programs within the community who can provide comprehensive drug and alcohol assessments is paramount, and clinicians are advised to establish lines for such referrals before the need actually arises. If the screening clinician has done the job correctly, resistance by the adolescent and his or her family will have been minimized. This increases the chances that referral will end up as a completed comprehensive assessment.

THE COMPREHENSIVE ASSESSMENT

The comprehensive assessment of an adolescent with a possible or likely SUD requires a broad view of the problems that predispose and maintain substance use and also those that commonly coexist with SUDs. Symptoms, behaviors, social context, and functioning within the multidomain context should all be examined. Although the emphasis will be primarily on substance use behaviors, a comprehensive assessment of adolescents with SUDs will not be altogether different from assessments for depression, anxiety, or other behavioral or emotional problems.

The Domain Model of Assessment

Substance use does not exist in a vacuum. There are multiple risk factors, frequent comorbidity, and multiple areas of possible dysfunction related to alcohol and other drug abuse. The comprehensive assessment of substance abuse and related problems requires evaluation of multiple areas of functioning in the adolescent's life and possible psychopathology. Over two decades ago, Tarter (1990) described a multilevel evaluation procedure for adolescents with suspected substance abuse. As shown in the adult literature and adult assessment instruments such as the Addiction Severity Index (McLellan, Luborsky, Woody, & O'Brien, 1980), the optimal assessment should not only assess substance use variables but also identify specific areas of dysfunction. Each of seven domains (see Table 4.1) should then be more thoroughly assessed by more detailed questions or by a standardized instrument designed to assess that specific domain.

TABLE 4.1. Domains of Assessment

- Substance use
  - Types of substances used
  - Onset
  - Pattern of use; frequency, quantity
- Psychiatric symptoms/disorders
  - Specific disorders
  - Onset
- Family functioning
  - Monitoring and supervision
  - Parental SUD, psychiatric disorders
  - Quality of parent–adolescent relationship
- School/vocational functioning
  - Current, recent grades; history of academic performance
  - Learning disorders; academic accommodations
  - School behavior
- Social competency/peer relations
  - Friends: quantity and quality
  - Level of peer deviance and substance use
  - Level of social skills
- Leisure/recreation
  - Access to and use of prosocial activities
  - Interests
- Medical
  - Chronic medical problems
  - Substance-induced problems

For both screening and more comprehensive assessments, examining a range of behaviors in addition to substance use is strongly recommended.

Once lifetime use of different substances has been determined (often in a previously administered screen), questions should become substance specific. If use of a particular substance is endorsed, the clinician should proceed with a more detailed inquiry about the frequency, quantity, negative consequences, context, and control of use for each specific substance. Despite the lower prevalence of the physical consequences of substance use (e.g., liver cirrhosis, alcohol withdrawal symptoms), questions about these features are essential. If answered in the affirmative, they indicate a severe level of substance dependency for the adolescent.

Developmentally Informed SUD Assessment

The clinician needs to conduct a developmentally informed assessment and be certain that adolescents (and family informants) understand each question. To increase the validity of symptom assessment in youth, it may be useful to provide a brief description of the symptom of interest to confirm that the teen and clinician have a common understanding of what is being asked. Providing the teen with specific examples of how the symptom may manifest in relation to the individual's developmental stage can facilitate recall of substance-related problems. Breaking questions down into component parts—that is, asking about one behavior at a time—may also improve the adolescent's understanding of symptom queries. Follow-up probes can help to clarify the context of symptom occurrence, thereby reducing false-positive symptoms.

For tolerance:

"Many kids tell me that they have to drink (use) more to get the same high or buzz. What about you?"

For withdrawal:

"Do you ever feel bad, get the shakes, sweats when you don't drink (use)? Especially after you have been using a lot for a while? Do you crave or really have to use to relieve these feelings?"

In addition, certain symptoms (e.g., physical tolerance to alcohol) need to be appropriately scaled to efficiently distinguish between normative and clinically significant levels of substance involvement in adolescents. For example, as adolescents adopt a somewhat regular pattern of binge drinking (generally daily or multiple times a week), their tolerance to alcohol may advance rapidly. Similarly, SUD symptoms may manifest differently in adolescents and adults owing to the developmental context in which the symptom occurs. Alternatively, some teens may interpret certain SUD symptoms in light of relatively limited experiences with substance use. Teens tend to endorse the symptom "drinking more or longer than intended" because of perceived social pressures to drink or because of inexperience with alcohol's effects; however, the intended interpretation of the symptom is a compulsion to engage in substance use.

Clinicians should consider expanding the assessment to include risky behaviors related to substance use such as sexual behavior, driving, fighting, or other activities with a potential for harm. In addition, the clinician should inquire about participation in the sale and distribution of illicit substances, diversion, and misuse of substances.

Substance Use Behavior

A comprehensive assessment of substance use should cover five major areas: (1) substances used, (2) patterns of use, (3) negative consequences, (4) context of use, and (5) control of use.

While quantity and frequency of use may suggest that an SUD is present, a DSM-5 SUD diagnosis requires use, impairment, and negative consequences of use and/or salient use behaviors.

The fifth edition of the American Psychiatric Association's (2013) *Diagnostic and Statistical Manual of Mental Disorders* (DSM-5) defines a single category of SUD for various substance classes using a set of 11 symptoms and requiring that two or more criteria be met before receiving an SUD diagnosis. It also has three severity levels—mild, moderate, and severe—based on the number of criteria endorsed. Some of DSM-5's symptoms are mild, developmentally normative for teenagers, and/or easily misunderstood and overendorsed. Those diagnosed may include many mild cases, which do not fit the classic definition of a compulsive pattern of substance use. This may unnecessarily apply a stigmatized and loaded label to youth whose problem severity may be mild and whose substance use pattern may be more intermittent than regular and more likely to remit (Winters, Martin, & Chung, 2011). The now discarded DSM-IV-TR (American Psychiatric Association, 2000) criterion of recurrent legal problems criteria led many adolescents to be diagnosed with abuse because they had gotten caught having or using substances rather than because of any specific problems with their use or pattern of use.

Two additional drug-related concepts are often confused with SUDs (Bukstein, 2007). Although not an official term, "misuse" can be defined as use for a purpose not consistent with medical guidelines (e.g., modifying dose, using to achieve euphoria, and/or using with other nonprescribed psychoactive substances). The term "diversion" refers to the transfer of medication from the individual for whom it was prescribed to one for whom it was not prescribed. While misuse and diversion are commonly noted with adolescents with SUDs, they are not synonymous with SUDs.

Specific Substances Used

Often building on a screen, the clinician asks not only about common substances—alcohol, marijuana, and tobacco—but also about less frequently used substances such as opiates, stimulants, steroids, and other prescription drugs. Questions should be specific. For example:

"Have you ever drunk a beer [or wine or hard liquor or mixed drinks]?"
"Have you ever used painkillers [specifically Vicodin, oxycodone]?"
"Have you ever used prescription drugs [more specifically stimulants such as Adderall or Ritalin or other 'ADHD drugs']?"
"Have you ever used downers [more specifically Xanax, Ativan, or Valium]?"

If the adolescent displays any indication of uncertainty or confusion, the clinician should provide specific examples, such as Vicodin or oxycodone for oral opiates. There are a variety of synthetic or "club" drugs that may not fit into any major drug category. These substances may be picked up by the question "Have you ever used any substance or drug to get high [or intoxicated] or to change your mood or thoughts?" Table 4.2 contains the major substance groups and some common street names. I advise clinicians to avoid slang, although many of the newer illicit substances are not commonly known by their chemical names. Street names and slang usually change too frequently for most clinicians to keep track of them. Attempts to be "cool" in hopes of furthering engagement often backfire.

Patterns of Use

When the adolescent endorses use of a substance, the clinician should explore patterns of use by asking about the types of agents used and the age of onset of use for each substance. In addition to age of first exposure and initial use, ask about the progression of use and the age at which the adolescent began regular use. Often, clinicians may be aware of quantity and/or frequency of use from their own screening of the teen. If this information is available from another clinician's screening, asking these questions again will serve as a reliability check and act as a more natural basis for asking about the other three major areas. While quantity and frequency data are essential to any complete assessment, the variability in adolescent substance use is often great. For example, binge drinking and increased substance use during weekends is quite common among adolescents rather than the often daily patterns seen in adults with SUDs. Therefore, the adolescent may report periods of abstinence as well as periods of rapid acceleration of use and heavy use of particular agents. The use of visual aids such as a time-line drug chart and calendar are often useful to allow the teen to report quantity, frequency, and variability data across time (usually past 30 days) with important dates, holidays, and other time cues as a guide. A specific form of this method, the time-line follow-back (TLFB), is used in research to obtain frequency of drug use within a previous specific interval (last week, last month, or last 90 days). The results from the TLFB are a common metric of SUD treatment outcome (i.e., percent or number of days of use or abstinence in the past 30 days).

Negative Consequences

Although reports of heavy alcohol or other drug use may be suggestive of a diagnosis of substance use disorder, an account of the negative

TABLE 4.2. Common Substances of Abuse

Name	Products and street names
Alcohol	Beer, wine, liquor
Cannabinoids	
Marijuana	Dope, grass, joint, weed, pot
Hashish	Hash, hemp
Nicotine (tobacco)	Cigarettes, cigars, snuff, spit, chew, e-cigarettes
Opioids	
Heroin	Smack, dope, H, white, horse
Opioids (oral)	Painkillers, oxycodone, OCs, Vicodin
Stimulants	
Cocaine	Coke, candy, crack, snow, blow, rock
Amphetamine/ methylphenidate/other stimulants	Bennies, speed, uppers, Adderall, Vyvanse, Concerta, Focalin, khat, methamphetamine (meth, ice, crystal, speed, crank)
Barbiturates/ other depressants	Downers, barbs, block busters, Christmas trees, goof balls, pinks, red devils, reds, and blues, and yellow jackets, GHB (easy lay, G), Rohypnol (roofies, rophies, ropies, roples, wolfies)
Benzodiazepines	Benzos, downers
Hallucinogens	
LSD	Acid, heaven, blotter
Mescaline	Buttons, mesc, peyote
Psilocybin	Magic mushrooms, shrooms
MDMA (methylenedioxy-methamphetamine)	Ecstasy, peace
K2/Spice, ketamine	Special K
Steroids	Juice, pumpers, roids, stackers, weight gainers
Other	Bath salts, dextromethorphan (DXM, dex), *Salvia divinorum*

consequences resulting from use is a cardinal sign of pathology in adolescents. Similar to screening, the clinician should be careful to inquire about directly related effects or negative consequences of use and not assume that all problems in an adolescent's life are due to substance use. In the comprehensive assessment, this inquiry is more detailed and asks specifically about negative consequences across domains (e.g., home, school, peer relations), with specific inquiry into their connection to substance use. Within the comprehensive assessment is a broader inquiry about functioning across domains, including mental health issues.

The clinician should also establish whether there is a pattern of use and negative consequences. Three or more times within a year is considered to be the minimum threshold for a pattern of behavior. Although this time line is somewhat arbitrary, it prevents one from identifying an SUD on the basis of cumulative lifeline consequences over several years. So, clinicians should ask how many times within a specific time period (e.g., the past year or 6 months), each of the events has occurred.

School

"Did your drinking/substance use cause you to get into significant trouble at school or cause you to break the rules at your school even if you were not caught?"

"Did your drinking/substance use cause you to quit school?"

If yes:

"Was the trouble you got in serious, such as getting expelled, suspended, or getting detention? How many times? Were the rules you broke serious ones, such as stealing or vandalism?"

"Did this rule breaking occur regularly for one month or more? Did this occur three times or more?"

Work

"Did using before or during work ever affect how you did on the job? Did you ever forget or were late for work?"

"Did your drinking/substance use cause serious problems at work, such as being demoted, getting fired, or having your supervisor threaten to fire you? Did you get fired because of anything you did while using or high?"

"What about a time when you were often intoxicated or very hungover while you were doing something important, like taking care of children? Or when you were supposed to be studying or going to school?"

Family

"What about missing something important, like family activities, because you were intoxicated or very hungover?"

"Did your drinking/substance use cause problems between you and your family members, or make existing problems much worse?"

"Were these problems significant and important, such as angry arguments, fights, or not talking to family members?"

"Did you ever drink/use substances in a situation in which it might have been dangerous to drink at all?"

"Did you ever drive while you were really too drunk to drive?"

"Did your drinking/substance use cause you to break (serious) laws?"

If yes:

"Were these illegal acts serious, such as stealing, vandalism, or drug dealing?"

"Were you ever arrested by the police because of something you did while drinking/using substances or while drunk?"

Peer Relations

"Did your drinking/other substance use cause problems between you and your friends or make existing problems much worse?"

"Were these problems significant and important, such as angry arguments, fights, or not talking to friends?"

"Did your drinking/other substance use cause problems between you and your girlfriend or boyfriend or make existing problems much worse?"

"Were these problems significant and important, such as angry arguments, fights, or not talking to your boyfriend or girlfriend?"

"Did your drinking/other substance use cause you to get into physical fights?"

Context of Use

The context of use includes the time and place of use; with whom use occurs; peer use levels, attitudes, and pressure; and information about who acquires the substance(s) to be used. Optimally, this assessment of context takes the form of a behavioral analysis of use with determination of the antecedents of use as well as the specific substance use behaviors and their consequences, both positive and negative. The adolescent's mood and attitude prior to and subsequent to use and his or her expectancies regarding use are also important elements in determining the overall social or substance-consuming milieu. For example:

"What does drinking or substance use do for you?"
"Why do you like it?"

The clinician should also inquire about the adolescent's values and attitudes in general. Does the adolescent possess nonconforming values, feel alienated from society, or have a sense of hopelessness about the world and his or her future in it? Assessment of substance use behavior may follow a functional analysis of use to determine usual antecedents to use and consequences of use. Such an analysis will allow a more specific targeting of relevant antecedents during treatment.

Control of Use

Has the adolescent tried to quit? Does he or she use more than planned? Does the teenager spend a lot of time using, being high or drunk, or being hungover? Is alcohol or another substance used in place of meeting role obligations such as going to school, doing schoolwork, working at a job, and spending time at hobbies or with family or friends? Does continued use cause significant physical or medical problems or make a physical or medical problem worse? Does the teen keep on drinking/using substances despite negative consequences? The continued use of alcohol or other substances despite the repeated occurrence of problems suggests an uncontrolled pattern of use. Questions designed to elicit SUD symptoms include the following.
     For withdrawal symptoms:

"Some people, after using alcohol or other drugs for a while, feel badly when they are not using; they may have the shakes (do you ever feel like this?), feel very anxious—or very depressed (do you ever feel like this?), be unable to sleep or sleep too much (has this happened to you?), or have extreme cravings to use the drug again?"

For the DSM-5 criterion of using more and longer than planned:

"Some people plan to not use drugs/or alcohol or maybe think that they will just use a bit, then end up using a lot more or for a longer period than they had originally planned."

For spending a lot of time planning to use, using, or recovering from use:

"Some people spend a lot—perhaps even most—of their time using substances. They may also spend a lot of time planning to use (buying and/or getting the means to buy) or recovering from using (e.g., a hangover or sleeping it off)—what about you? How many hours a day all together do you spend using, planning to use, or recovering from use?"

For craving:

"How often do you think about using [drugs] with the thought that you would really like to use, really want to use?"

For tolerance:

"Does it take more [drinks, joints, pills] to get you high/drunk/get a buzz? How much more—twice as much, four times as much? How many more?"

Several other areas of inquiry are not covered by the DSM-5 criteria but deserve attention. Blackouts during use, especially alcohol use, can be thought of as a negative consequence and one that often bothers the adolescent, perhaps setting the stage for increasing motivation for treatment. Another question is whether friends or family have expressed concern about the teenager's use.

Throughout the interview, the clinician should elicit the adolescent's attitude or feelings about his or her answers: "What do you think/feel about that?"

Treatment History

A past history of interventions for SUDs is not uncommon in adolescents who have been using substances for a few years or more. Create an inventory of each episode of assessment and treatment: its onset (including relevant precipitants), duration, type of modalities utilized, outcome, and the adolescent's and parent's perception of its value.

Other Domains

I have focused on the substance use domain in this chapter, although additional inquiry should be made within other domains listed in Figure 4.3. Particularly important are symptoms of other mental health problems such as depression and other mood disorders, anxiety disorders, trauma history and symptoms of posttraumatic stress disorder (PTSD), ADHD, conduct disorder (including aggression, criminal activity, and legal history), oppositional–defiant behavior, psychosis, and eating disorders. The relationship of symptoms of psychiatric disorders to the onset and exacerbation of substance use and other problems should add critical information to the assessment. Regardless of the response to the questions about symptoms or behaviors, the clinician should ask about any current or past mental health treatment history (including visits to therapists, psychologists, and/or psychiatrists). Additionally, the clinician should ask both the teen and parents about current and past medications for behavioral or emotional difficulties. Questions about suicidal history are mandatory, including hopelessness, ideation, intent, plan, and past attempts. Positive answers to screening questions should be followed by a more comprehensive mental health evaluation or referral to a mental health provider or facility as soon as possible.

The remaining domains (family functioning, leisure activities, peer relationships, academic functioning, and medical problems) provide a baseline for the level of overall functioning and help determine whether substance use has been adversely affecting any specific domain(s).

Inquiry into the family, peer, and school domains often presents as questions related to risk factor status and should be asked of both teen and parent.

"What is life like at your home? What do you do together—do you enjoy it, or is it a chore, painful? Do you get along with your folks? Do you spend time together? Do your parents know where you go when you are not at home or school? Do they ask about where you are going, or do they know where you are going? Do you have a curfew? Do they know about your alcohol/drug use? Do you think they care? Do your parents use alcohol or other drugs?"

"Tell me about your friends. What do you do with your friends? Do you wish you had more friends, better friends? Do your parents like your friends? Have they ever met your friends? Do any of your friends use alcohol or other drugs? Do you think they have a problem? Do they think you have a problem?"

Additional peer questions should center around the presence of romantic interests and sexual behavior, including high-risk sexual behavior (multiple partners, no condom use).

"Tell me about school. Where do you go? What grade level? Do you get any special help at school, or are you in any special programs? How are you doing in school? Your grades? What kind of grades have you made? Are you satisfied by your grades? Your school effort? Do you want to do better? Can you do better?"

The school domain also includes questions about work history. What jobs has the teen had? How long did he or she work? Was he or she ever fired? The medical domain should include questions about general health status and any recent medical treatments, including medications, allergies, and past and recent accidents. Finally, the recreational domains consist of questions about what the adolescent does in his or her free time, including substance use and behaviors associated with use and prosocial activities such as athletics, video gaming, and other computer use.

Aside from an emphasis on the substance use domain, comprehensive assessment for SUDs should not greatly differ from comprehensive assessment for other mental health problems in adolescents.

The Use of Instruments for a Comprehensive Assessment

The value of standardized instruments to the clinician includes their ability to obtain more consistent, reliable information to complement clinical interviews; to obtain comparable measures at regular intervals; and to define more homogeneous patient populations to determine treatment needs. Instruments can help determine relevant outcome variables, be an adjunct to clinical judgment, and potentially offer the user a less expensive and more efficient method of assessment. An increased emphasis on reporting the outcomes of our interventions has led to an increased interest in using instruments.

Whether the user is a clinician or a researcher, the attributes of a good instrument are the same. The instrument should be valid; that is, it should measure the concept it purports to measure. The instrument should be reliable; that is, it should be consistent in its results across time and across users. Finally, the instrument should be practical; it should not demand too much time, effort, or cost for the amount and type of information it provides.

Several major types of instruments are used in the assessment of adolescents with suspected or confirmed problems with substance use. While I have attempted to be as complete as possible, the dynamic nature of instrument development means that there may be newer instruments, and more recent versions of more established instruments, than what I have included.

Comprehensive Instruments

The use of multiple instruments for the assessment of adolescents is not always practical for clinical programs. The search for a single comprehensive instrument or group of complementary instruments to assess adolescent substance use and related problems has led to the development of several such instruments. Examples of comprehensive assessment instruments, usually delivered as an interview, include the T-ASI (Kaminer et al., 1993) and GAIN (Dennis et al., 1998). Some individuals or programs use instruments designed for prevention, such as the DUSI and POSIT, as part of their comprehensive assessment. Other examples of comprehensive instruments include the Adolescent Diagnostic Interview and the CDDR. The clinician or researcher should consider the use of other instruments to augment substance use assessment procedures.

Experienced, trained clinicians can administer semistructured diagnostic instruments or interviews that generated specific psychiatric diagnoses, including SUDs. Perhaps the best known of these diagnostic instruments is the Schedule for Affective Disorders and Schizophrenia for School-Age Children (K-SADS; Kaufman et al., 2016). Particularly in cases with substantial psychiatric-SUD comorbidity, the K-SADS provides a review of specific diagnostic criteria and chronology for the onset of symptoms that may assist the clinician in understanding the relationship between comorbid diagnoses. Martin and colleagues (1995) modified the DSM-III-R version of the SCID to specifically assess DSM-IV substance use disorders among adolescents. Symptoms and diagnoses showed good concurrent validity and moderate to good interrater reliability (Martin, Pollock, Bukstein, & Lynch, 2000).

Other Instruments

Practical administration of instruments is a primary concern. Valuable time should not be taken up in the assessment of variables that are not needed or will not be used in targeting treatment interventions within the treatment program.

Too often, clinicians equate assessment with obtaining baseline information. They forget that assessment continues throughout treatment and beyond. Outcomes assessment usually consists of variables related to quantity and frequency of substance use. Clinicians should also consider gathering measures of global impairment or specific measures related to any critical mediating variables such as family functioning. The prevalence of adolescents with comorbid psychiatric disorders dictates that outcome also includes dimensional measures of psychopathology, such as conduct disorder, ADHD, depression, or anxiety. The TLFB methodology can provide a daily tabulation of drinking and substance use behavior during the previous month or 90-day period, providing a quantity and frequency assessment both through the course of the intervention and at designated follow-up points (Maisto, Connors, & Allen, 1995; Waldron et al., 2001). The TLFB results are expressed as days drug free or, conversely, days of drug use per interval (week, month, etc.). Finally, urine drug screens are often the singular method for following abstinence outcomes but are unable to demonstrate nonabstinent substance use improvements or improvement in functioning, either globally or within specific domains. Increasing demands from third-party payors for evidence of outcomes should motivate clinicians to regularly conduct outcome assessments.

SUMMARY

Screening and assessment are the foundation of clinical intervention for adolescents with SUDs, determining who should be treated, what problems exist, and ultimately the effectiveness of treatment. Clinicians should develop a level of competence with interview and instrument use commensurate with the demands of their roles in dealing with adolescents. Because of the common presence of multiple problems in teens with SUDs, I advocate for screening and assessment across a broad range of life domains, utilizing a combination of face-to-face interviews and instruments with sound psychometric properties. Finally, assessment continues through, and even following, acute treatment in order to ascertain the effects of interventions.

Chapter Five

Treatment Planning and Brief Interventions

After an adolescent has been appropriately assessed, the next step is to select an intervention. Selection depends on a number of factors. Particularly important is access to treatment that includes the availability of trained professionals with expertise and experience in treating adolescents with SUDs. In this chapter, I discuss how clinicians, adolescents, and their families make decisions about which interventions to use. This discussion includes general elements of optimal SUD treatment and levels of care, and it concludes with an overview of brief interventions.

WHO CAN TREAT ADOLESCENTS WITH SUDs?

To provide developmentally appropriate treatment for youth, clinicians need a background in the developmental tasks of adolescents and the salient risk factors that can sometimes cause a typical trajectory to go awry. Development is also affected by social media and other cultural influences. Without an understanding of typical development and the myriad ways it can be impacted by cultural, familial, social, and other outside forces, it is impossible to provide informed treatment to children and teens under the influence.

I have used the term "clinician" throughout this book to refer to all professionals who work with youth. Admittedly, not all professionals will assume each of the potential roles involved in assessment and treatment, but all must be cognizant of the elements of effective treatment in order to support the systems, providers, and policies that deal with adolescents with SUDs. These systems include health care, behavioral health (psychiatric and SUD treatment), schools, juvenile justice, and public welfare. In each of these systems, professionals deal with youth with substance use and SUDs, albeit from slightly different perspectives and different roles. Professionals in all of these separate systems should be acquainted with screening content and procedures. Fewer will develop skills in comprehensive assessment, although those in the behavioral health field who deal with adolescents should have basic skills in this area. Similarly, clinicians in the behavioral health field should have a fairly high level of comfort in dealing with such youth. If they cannot provide appropriate levels of assessment and treatment, they should at least have knowledge of what interventions might be appropriate and where to access such treatments and providers to deliver them.

Referral to Treatment

Teens who are not willing or able to engage in a brief intervention should be referred either to an allied mental health professional (such as a social worker, psychologist, or other counselor in the primary care setting) or to a substance abuse treatment program appropriate for adolescents for further support. Appropriate substance abuse treatment programs for adolescents should be scientifically based, family oriented, and developmentally appropriate. Professionals involved with adolescents should be aware of community resources and have established referral patterns to specific programs or professionals who provide SUD treatment for adolescents.

ELEMENTS OF EFFECTIVE TREATMENT

Despite the identification of effective treatments for adolescents with SUDs, a substantial proportion of youth do not respond to specific treatments. Currently, there are no empirical results that can guide us in matching specific treatment modalities with specific types of adolescents. Nevertheless, based on the combination of empirical research and current clinical consensus, clinicians dealing with adolescents with SUDs should develop a treatment plan that ideally includes:

- Motivation and engagement (see Chapter 2).
- Family involvement to improve supervision, monitoring, and communication between parents and adolescent (see Chapters 7 and 8).
- Improved problem-solving skills, social skills, and relapse prevention (see Chapter 6).
- Comorbid psychiatric disorders through psychosocial treatments and/or medication (see Chapter 9).
- Increasing prosocial behaviors, peer relationships, and academic functioning (see Chapter 6).
- Adequate duration of treatment, including provision of follow-up care following acute treatment.

Self-help support groups can be encouraged as adjuncts to these modalities. These critical elements of treatment for adolescents with SUDs are an abbreviated version of "Principles of Adolescent Substance Use Disorder Treatment," recently developed by the National Institute on Drug Abuse (NIDA; 2014). These principles are listed in Table 5.1 and are based on research evidence.

Most clinicians support achieving and maintaining abstinence from substance use as the primary goal of treatment of adolescents with SUDs. While abstinence may be the explicit goal of treatment, a more nuanced and perhaps realistic view recognizes the chronicity of SUDs in some populations of youth and the self-limited nature of problem substance use and substance use–related problems in others. The majority of posttreatment adolescents improve in overall functioning and decrease their substance use without maintaining abstinence, and so harm reduction may be a reasonable interim, implicit goal of treatment. Harm reduction proposes, as a goal, reduction in the use and adverse effects of substances, a reduction in the severity and frequency of relapses, and improvement in one or more domains of the adolescent's functioning (e.g., academic performance or family functioning) without necessarily achieving abstinence from all substances of abuse. Adolescents may not be initially motivated to stop substance use or able to accept the notion of lifelong abstinence. However, learning skills to deal with problematic substance use may provide the adolescent with greater self-efficacy to not only reduce use but also ultimately move toward abstinence if abstinence works for that adolescent. In addition, the clinician clears the road for eventual recovery from the consequences of SUDs and potentially toward a substance-free lifestyle by targeting risk factors for SUDs such as parental monitoring, parent–adolescent conflict, deviant peers, and lack of prosocial activities. Improvements in psychosocial functioning may prompt greater

TABLE 5.1. NIDA Principles of Adolescent SUD Treatment

1. Adolescent substance use needs to be identified and addressed as soon as possible.

2. Adolescents can benefit from a drug abuse intervention even if they are not addicted to a drug.

3. Routine annual medical visits are an opportunity to ask adolescents about drug use.

4. Legal interventions and sanctions or family pressure may play an important role in getting adolescents to enter, stay in, and complete treatment.

5. Substance use disorder treatment should be tailored to the unique needs of the adolescent.

6. Treatment should address the needs of the whole person rather than just focusing on his or her drug use.

7. Behavioral therapies are effective in addressing adolescent drug use.

8. Families and the community are important aspects of treatment.

9. Effectively treating substance use disorders in adolescents requires also identifying and treating any other mental health conditions they may have.

10. Sensitive issues such as violence and child abuse or risk of suicide should be identified and addressed.

11. It is important to monitor drug use during treatment.

12. Staying in treatment for an adequate period of time and continuity of care afterward are important.

13. Testing adolescents for sexually transmitted diseases like HIV, as well as hepatitis B and C, is an important part of drug treatment.

Note. From NIDA (2014).

appreciation for prosocial behavior; more optimal social, family, and academic functioning; and the real or potential costs of continued substance use. Although harm reduction may be an interim implicit goal of treatment, controlled use of any nonprescribed substance of abuse should be avoided as an explicit goal in the treatment of adolescents. Tolerance of substance use in an adolescent being treated for SUDs is different from appearing to prescribe substance use.

Control of substance use (i.e., abstinence or reduced use) should rarely be the only goal of treatment. As a broad concept, rehabilitation involves targeting associated problems and domains of functioning. Integrated interventions that concurrently deal with coexisting psychiatric and behavioral problems, family functioning, peer and interpersonal relationships, and academic and vocational functioning not only should produce general improvement in psychosocial functioning, but they are also more likely to yield improved outcomes in the primary treatment goal of achieving and maintaining control of substance use. The risk factors within the domain model of assessment (see Table 4.1) provide targets for treatment. As discussed in Chapter 1, the majority of evidence-based models of treatment of adolescents with SUDs involve family interventions, and some, such as multisystemic therapy (MST), also address extrafamilial risk factors.

Admittedly, offering a potentially broad treatment menu may be a difficult task for individual professionals. They often have limited training and resources, and programs may have similar problems providing comprehensive treatment across multiple modalities. Clinicians cannot do everything at once, nor are adolescents and their families often amenable to extended interventions. Triage decisions must be made about the importance of problems and the sequence of interventions. Particularly in cases involving moderate to severe comorbid psychiatric disorders, clinicians can disagree about what problem to address first. Even when substance use is the identified problem, the lack of attention to other problems that may reinforce substance use may complicate substance abuse treatment.

The general rule of thumb is to treat the problem that has the most immediate impact on functioning and/or presents the most immediate danger to the adolescent or others. In many, if not most, cases, intervention for substance use will be first, but there are notable exceptions— suicidal behavior, psychosis, severe aggressive behavior with injury or potential for serious injury to others, and uncontrolled eating disorder. Most of these exceptions seem obvious; the more difficult issue is to determine when to introduce SUD intervention(s) or, in the case of SUD treatment first, when to start treatment on the comorbid psychiatric disorder. The prevailing model remains sequential treatment with SUD treatment first, then psychiatric treatment.

There are several problems with this sequential model. The first and perhaps most important one is the effect that untreated or inadequately treated psychiatric problems have on SUD treatment success (and vice versa). My motivation for entering this field was my dissatisfaction with the dichotomous treatment model in which adolescents who more often than not have significant comorbid disorders cannot be or were not treated under one roof. A second problem is more practical. Teens and parents are unlikely to tolerate extended, intensive treatment episodes, especially across different settings and/or providers, and third-party payors are very reluctant to pay for such episodes. In other words, we usually have a limited amount of time and resources to treat each adolescent. Some type of integrated or concurrent treatment seems to be the best goal for adolescents with psychiatric comorbidity.

RESPONDING TO PARENT CONCERNS

Following assessment, the clinician reports to the adolescent and parents. Common parent questions, with suggested responses, are as follows.

1. *Question:* "Does my child need treatment?"

   Answer: "If your child displays a pattern of drug and/or alcohol use that results in impairment, some level of intervention should be provided."

2. *Question:* "What kind of treatment does he or she need?"

   Answer: "The best type of treatment for your adolescent and family depends on several factors: his or her motivation to change behavior, any identified risk factors such as peer influence, family conflict, adequacy of parental monitoring and supervision, signs of severe physical addiction such as withdrawal symptoms, and the presence of other psychiatric disorders such as depression and ADHD."

3. *Question:* "Do we send him or her to rehab?"

   Answer: "Adolescents should be treated in the least restrictive environment. Previous treatment failures at lower levels of care may dictate inpatient or residential treatment. However, some type of community-based treatment will be necessary when the teen returns from such a program."

4. *Question:* "Can we force him or her into treatment?"

   Answer: "Perhaps 'force' is not the best word to use. However, you, the school, and the juvenile justice system can provide sanctions if your child does not follow through on assessment recommendations. You can use your adolescent's privileges, such as car or cell phone use, as an incentive for treatment participation and removal for nonparticipation."

5. *Question:* "What if my child has a psychiatric problem?"

   Answer: "Coexisting psychiatric problems should be identified and treated with evidence-based treatments, either integrated into substance use treatment or run concurrently with it."

Choosing a Treatment Program

While the assessing clinician makes treatment recommendations, discussed in more detail below, the ultimate selection of a treatment program or provider is usually made by parents based on their preferences and resources, including health insurance. Parents should ask prospective treatment programs about the following:

> "How is the most appropriate and least restrictive level of care determined?"
>
> "How many levels of care do you have? What determines the level at which my teen is treated?"
>
> "What therapeutic activities are involved? For my child? For us?"
>
> "What is the experience and training of the professional staff?"
>
> "Does the program use evidence-based treatment modalities? What are they?"
>
> "If my child has a psychiatric problem, how is this problem assessed and treated?"
>
> "How long is the program, and on what does its duration depend?"

The next section outlines the possible levels of care for adolescents with substance use problems and discusses which levels may be appropriate for specific adolescents.

LEVELS OF CARE

Treatment of adolescents with SUDs can take place at one of several levels of care, reflecting intensity of treatment and restriction of movement. These levels range from large-scale prevention efforts in school-based groups or media campaigns through brief treatment, more sustained outpatient care, intensive outpatient interventions, and, finally, residential treatment of variable duration. Factors affecting the choice of treatment setting, or level of care, include the following:

1. The need to provide a safe environment and the ability of the adolescent to care for him- or herself.
2. Motivation and willingness of the adolescent and his or her family to cooperate with treatment.
3. The adolescent's need for structure and limit setting that cannot be provided in a less restrictive environment.
4. The existence of additional medical or psychiatric conditions that require additional high-level professional staff or consultation.
5. The availability of specific types of treatment settings for adolescents.
6. The adolescent's and his or her family's preferences for a particular setting.
7. Treatment failure in a less restrictive setting or level of care.

Although residential programs, such as therapeutic communities, have a place in the range of setting options, community intervention settings, if feasible, may offer optimal generalization of treatment gains. Even in the community, alternative sites of intervention, such as home and school, are being used.

For the clinician, initial placement decisions most often depend on acute or presenting status. Medical or psychiatric status often dictates the level of care. For example, the need for medical detoxification (in the case of opiate, benzodiazepine, or high and persistent alcohol use) may require the use of an inpatient setting such as a detoxification or psychiatric unit or a specialized outpatient detoxification program. The presence or suspicion of a high level of psychiatric symptoms such as psychosis and suicidal and/or homicidal behavior, particularly in the presence of uncontrolled substance use by an adolescent, often dictates inpatient psychiatric assessment and treatment. Although these psychiatric problems usually "stand alone" as reasons for inpatient admission (usually to psychiatric programs), the presence of high levels of substance use will often reduce the threshold for admission to inpatient or acute residential treatment. Although SUDs merit consideration in inpatient psychiatric admission and discharge decisions, generally, these decisions are made on the basis of psychiatric or medical concerns—danger to self or others, poor reality testing and clouded sensorium (i.e., psychosis), and medical instability (e.g., withdrawal symptoms, eating disorders).

Although the stated reason for psychiatric admission of adolescents with SUDs will be psychiatric symptoms and impairment, psychiatric inpatient admission potentially offers a teachable moment that can increase the adolescent's motivation to seek specific or integrated SUD treatment.

The American Society of Addiction Medicine (ASAM; 2013) developed a set of placement criteria to guide decisions related to clinically appropriate placement decisions of adolescents. It complements a similar set of placement criteria for adults. The criteria read as a matrix, with various levels of care from I to IV and sublevels distinguished by medical support or level of supervision. Placement in the various levels depends on the severity reached by each patient in six dimensions: (1) intoxication and/or withdrawal potential; (2) biomedical conditions or complications; (3) emotional, behavioral, or cognitive complications as indicated by dangerousness/lethality, interference with addiction recovery efforts, social functioning, ability for self-care, and course of illness; (4) readiness to change; (5) relapse, continued use, or continued problem potential; and (6) recovery environment. Each level of placement (I, II, III, or IV) needs to be supported by a level of severity (rating of 0–4 points) in the various dimensions. The actual application of the placement criteria can be complicated. Real-life placements are limited by the availability and quality of the programs representing each of the levels' and sublevels' placement criteria, trained staff who can deliver services within the model specified by the placement criteria, and finally, third-party payors who support the criteria and will pay for treatment at each level of care. Nevertheless, many states make Medicaid payments, and some commercial payors make reimbursement contingent upon meeting the ASAM placement criteria. The ASAM criteria have face validity, meaning they make sense to most clinicians as a basis for placement decisions. However, the criteria are supported by surprisingly little data. It's unclear whether placement according to the criteria results in optimal outcomes. Nevertheless, the criteria provide clinicians with a framework for trying to make these decisions.

Most placements in higher levels of care are based on failure at lower levels of care. Evidence of failure can include continued substance use and negative consequences, relapse, lack of compliance, and environmental problems preventing the successful use of a lower level of care. Starting with outpatient or intensive outpatient levels of care seems reasonable at least for an initial treatment episode. Exceptions might include the presence of significant withdrawal and the need for medical detoxification. At a lower level of care, the clinician will be able to test motivation, compliance, and acute response to treatment. Problems with these areas of treatment can result in modifications in level of care.

Residential versus Community-Based Treatment

Decades ago, residential treatment for 28 days or more was the prevailing setting for adolescent SUD treatment. The primary goal was to take adolescents out of their environment (marked by drug-using peers, cues related to substance use, and stressors) that was contributing to the development and maintenance of substance use. At the time, there were insufficient community-based alternatives, with few, if any, evidence-based outpatient modalities available. Today, the availability of evidence-based, community-based modalities allows for potentially effective outpatient therapy, a less intensive level of care. The primary value of residential treatment is its ability to control the adolescent's environment when he or she is unable or unwilling to control substance use. This inability to control or attenuate use must now be evidenced at a lower level of care for residential care to be considered. Even with successful residential treatment, the adolescent will return to the community and to those aspects of the environment that prompted or maintained the substance use. In this home environment, community-based treatment must consolidate any residential gains and maintain them. Family and peer issues, from which the adolescent was protected in residential care, become paramount. In other words, the real treatment usually begins back in the community.

BRIEF INTERVENTIONS

Assessment, treatment planning, and intervention with adolescents with substance use and SUDs intersect at brief interventions (BIs). Brief interventions typically consist of one to four sessions. They can be stand-alone interventions or the beginning of ongoing care that could include any evidence-based treatment such as CBT or family approaches (Center for Substance Abuse Treatment, 1999a). Almost always, BIs for adolescents with SUDs include a motivational component, which may emphasize increasing motivation for the adolescent's choice of abstinence, or motivation to participate in a more intensive level of treatment. The motivational component is useful for adolescents on waiting lists and schools, and for primary health care settings as part of screening, brief intervention, and referral to treatment (SBIRT; Tait & Hulse, 2003).

Learning to apply BIs is a valuable skill for a wide range of clinicians, especially those outside the formal SUD treatment community who may not be able to be part of a large SUD treatment program but see a range of adolescents who use substances and may or may not have an SUD. BIs can consist of feedback from assessment and treatment planning for SUD treatment because both feedback and treatment planning help to prepare adolescents not to use, to use less, or to stop using substances.

Since motivation is usually a major component of a BI, it is not surprising that an MI approach is used in almost all existing BI protocols. My description of MI in Chapter 2 follows the outline of behavior change counseling. A quick BI is brief advice, which usually takes not more than 5–15 minutes in a health care professional's office. It uses expert feedback to communicate risk while demonstrating respect. Behavioral change counseling is a more substantial BI; in addition to feedback and advice, the clinician attempts to establish rapport and uses MI strategies based on adolescent readiness to set an agenda for change and build motivation for that change.

Key Characteristics of BIs

Bien et al. (1993) describe several important characteristics of effective BIs using the acronym FRAMES: feedback, responsibility, advice, menu, empathy, and self-efficacy. Note that the FRAMES components are not listed in chronological order of likely use.

■ **Feedback.** From assessment of current status. Using an objective, noncoercive presentation, the clinician provides personalized information about the problem behavior (substance use and its effects). The clinician offers factual details about the adolescent's substance use, use patterns in comparison with norms for use in similar-age peer groups, and information about substance use risk and harms from use. The clinician then asks the adolescent for feedback about the feedback: "What do you make of this?" or "How does this fit or not fit with what you know about yourself?"

■ **Responsibility.** Personal decision to change. Adolescents value autonomy, and the clinician emphasizes the adolescent's freedom of choice: "It's your choice when you are ready"; "It's up to you; you're free to decide to change or not"; "No one else can really decide for you or force you to change."

■ **Advice.** Recommend behavior change. As an extension to the simple intervention of giving information to the adolescent, the clinician offers clear recommendations on the need to change substance use behaviors. The clinician uses a supportive, concerned tone. Advice on specific ways to change substance use should be preceded by asking permission: "Is it OK if I go over with you what options you have?"

■ **Menu.** Create a selection of treatment options. The clinician attempts to elicit intervention options from the adolescent, and if the adolescent is unable to provide them, the clinician asks permission to provide a variety of treatment options that the adolescent may consider. Considering a menu of options essentially constitutes the beginning of treatment planning, although the focus is enlisting the adolescent's input about treatment. Choosing from a menu reinforces autonomy and the idea that the adolescent has some choice; teens cannot be made to pursue a particular treatment, or even treatment in general, if they truly do not want to. The menu should consist of options that are acceptable to parents. Discussion with parents can be included in a BI model.

■ **Empathy.** Be supportive and understanding about the adolescent's situation. In a supportive, nonjudgmental manner, the clinician uses techniques such as affirmations, reflections, and summaries to convey an understanding of the adolescent's subjective experience. The clinician acknowledges the difficulty of addressing the problems of substance use as well as any perceived benefits from substance use that the adolescent would be giving up: "Quitting is tough"; "You've made a lot of hard decisions and changes in your life."

■ **Self-efficacy.** Reinforce hope and optimism. The clinician optimistically supports the adolescent's belief that he or she can successfully tackle changing substance use behaviors. Together, the adolescent and clinician attempt to identify past successes and reframe prior failures as lessons learned: "I know that when you are ready you will be able to do this";

"I know you have learned a lot about the kinds of things that can trip you up"; "You have been able to stay clean for quite a while in the past."

A Change Plan

Although not part of the FRAMES acronym, discussion of a change plan should be the result of following the FRAMES elements. After summarizing reasons for changing substance use or other behavior(s), the clinician and adolescent set goals for change, consider options, outline specific steps (what the adolescent will do and when), identify potential obstacles and how they might be overcome, and show how the adolescent and others will evaluate his or her progress. A change plan is a summary of MI and BI efforts. An example of a change plan follows.

CLINICIAN: Bill, after realizing how much you are drinking and its effect on your mood, you are telling me that you would like to address these issues.

ADOLESCENT: Yeah.

CLINICIAN: I have a piece of paper here, and on it I am writing these specific goals: (1) reduce drinking and (2) improve mood. Now what can we do to achieve these goals? Let's start with drinking. Do you have any ideas about what might help you achieve these goals?

ADOLESCENT: I'm not sure. I do know that I drink when I am bored.

CLINICIAN: OK, that's a start—it sounds like you may need to plan your activities better so that you have less free, unstructured time. For example, many kids find it useful to go out with friends only if they have a planned, positive activity with their friends and not just hanging out.

ADOLESCENT: Yes, but sometimes, even after going to a movie, a concert, or playing ball; we are back at the house. I guess when that happens, I usually don't make good decisions—it's too late.

CLINICIAN: That's pretty common in my experience. If you like, I can tell you about a type of therapy that helps kids problem solve around such high-risk situations for using.

ADOLESCENT: Sure.

CLINICIAN: It's called CBT, or cognitive-behavioral therapy. CBT can even be used in groups or individually. I will help identify triggers for use or high-risk situations and what you can do if you find yourself in those situations.

ADOLESCENT: I think that sounds like what I might need. I would like the group.

CLINICIAN: OK. A few more questions. How will we know if this is working? And how will we track this?

ADOLESCENT: I guess I will be drinking less. I hope my life—school and fighting with my parents—gets better.

CLINICIAN: Yes, we can track your school attendance and grades and ask both you and your parents how you are communicating and following the rules. Hopefully, you can let us know how much you are drinking. Finally, what are the potential obstacles for completing your plan, and how will you deal with these obstacles?

A Flexible BI Model

A BI model for adolescent SUDs is flexible, with sessions ranging from one to four depending on the level of adolescent engagement, motivation, readiness for change, self-efficacy, progress through the stages of BI tasks, and need for more intensive ongoing treatment. If the adolescent progresses from one stage to another rapidly (e.g., becomes ready to discuss a change plan in the first session), the clinician should follow the teen's lead. The following outlines the possible content of a four-session BI.

SESSION 1: FEEDBACK AND ENHANCE MOTIVATION

- Objective, nonjudgmental feedback about problem(s).
- Use of OARS strategies (see Chapter 2) to increase change talk.
- Elicit adolescent comments about the problem, reasons for change, need for change, and intention to change.

CLINICIAN: Sally, we have reviewed your drug use and how that compares to what most kids your age are—or are not—doing. What do you think? [open question]

ADOLESCENT: I know that I am using a lot—a lot more than I should. I guess I would be better off by quitting. But what would I do? All my friends use.

CLINICIAN: You are really worried about what would replace drug use in your life. You might be lonely and without any friends. But you seem like you feel that many parts of your life would be better without drugs. That's a tough trade-off. [double-sided reflection]

ADOLESCENT: Yeah. I have some nonusing friends, but I don't know if they would want to hang out with a druggie.

CLINICIAN: You seen like a resourceful, bright young lady. What ideas can you think of to replace your drug-using friends? [affirmation, open question]

SESSION 2: CHANGE PLAN

- Review and summarize reasons for change (decreasing substance use).
- Consider change options.
- Develop the plan.
  - Steps: What will the client do and when?
  - Support: Who will be there to support change, and how will they provide the support?
  - Obstacles: Anticipate obstacles and how they will be overcome.
  - Signs of progress: How will the adolescent know that what he or she is doing is working and that goals are being met?
- Elicit adolescent comments about the plan.

SESSION 3: RECOVERY SKILLS

- Review progress during BI, including change plan.
- Discuss triggers for use and plan to deal with triggers.
- Plan for crises and emergencies.
- Consider obstacles and resources.
- Elicit adolescent comments.

SESSION 4: BOOSTER AND/OR PARENT SESSION

Booster Sessions (to enhance motivation and check on the change plan)

- Review progress.
- Address difficulties in implementing the change plan.
- Review (as needed) recovery skills (see Chapter 6).
- Consider the need for more intensive intervention.

Parent Session

- Review adolescent change plan and progress.
- Parent monitoring and supervision, communication, contracts, and CM (see Chapter 7).

Summary of BIs

BIs offer a flexible alternative to longer, more intensive interventions for adolescents with SUDs. They focus on enhancing motivation for change, developing a change plan, and, when needed, providing a succinct introduction to recovery skills. BIs are an important option for professions dealing with adolescents who use substances. While designed to be delivered in primary care medical settings, BIs also have potential to be used in schools or by mental health clinicians. They can serve as stand-alone interventions, especially for teens with less severe substance use presentations, or as preparation for more intensive intervention.

OUTPATIENT TREATMENT

Outpatient intervention usually consists of a single modality such as family, group, or individual therapy, with a frequency of one or perhaps two times a week. Both the limited intensity and specific modality present constraints, especially in cases where the adolescent has many problems and there are multiple potential targets for therapy. Attempting to combine family and individual therapy may dilute the intensity. Clinicians need to respect the time constraints of families and may need to work with them on a treatment plan that focuses on limited targets such as providing motivation and relapse prevention for individual therapy and establishing appropriate limits and family problem solving for family therapy. All of the evidence-based practices discussed in Chapter 1 are outpatient modalities.

Specific treatment models may be differentially efficacious for particular subgroups of youth and/or may be associated with different patterns of outcomes across different domains of functioning. For example, more resistant adolescents may be better served by family therapy, and those more motivated may benefit more from CBT. More resistant youth may need some MI-based intervention and/or contingency management, whereas others may be ready for skills-based modalities without additional motivation-based interventions. More research is needed to identify which adolescents may be more likely to respond to specific kinds of interventions in order to meet the specific needs and deficits of adolescents—or to capitalize on their strengths. Until these questions of the best individualized plan involving specific or combination of interventions have been addressed more adequately, clinicians have the flexibility to choose from among the well-established treatments, depending on how the approaches fit within their current treatment environments and staffing resources.

The interventions listed in Chapter 1 and in later chapters represent a limited number of the total types of treatments used for adolescents with SUDs. Many other treatments may be effective and some not. Adoption of evidence-based practices may be limited by the resources necessary to train and supervise staff as well as time and program philosophy considerations. While we do not know enough about the active elements of evidence-based practices to separate aspects of these practices or evidence-based practice and apply them to a system of adolescent-treatment matching (i.e., which evidence-based practice will result in the best outcomes for specific adolescents), I encourage clinicians to adopt what they can from evidence-based practices, if not the practices themselves.

INTENSIVE OUTPATIENT TREATMENT

Intensive outpatient care provides an intensive experience in a community setting. In a group format, adolescents are exposed to a combination of modalities that may vary widely by program. Usually, there are three sessions per week, for about 9 hours a week. Adolescents receive psycho-education and participate in process-oriented, skills-oriented groups that might include CBT, MET, and dialectical behavior therapy (DBT). Some programs might add multiple family groups with psychoeducational or process content. In addition to the groups, therapists may meet with the adolescent and family individually. The duration of the programs varies from 2 to 8 weeks. Although the content varies from program to program, many programs have advanced from a traditional 12-step focus to include more structured evidence-based practices and therapeutic activities, including CBT. I cannot stress enough the need for structure, consistency, and interventions based on evidence-based methods. Twelve-step–oriented programs are discussed later in this chapter.

RESIDENTIAL LEVELS OF CARE

Questions about the effectiveness of residential settings remain, including generalization of improvements back to the community, the common absence of substantial family involvement in treatment, and cost effectiveness, especially relative to other less intensive or less expensive community-based alternatives. The active ingredients in such interventions may be removal from a problem environment, maturity, and efforts to keep the adolescent busy. The development of more adaptive social skills may be either an overt or inadvertent goal. Many programs suggest that program graduates may need longer-term therapeutic boarding schools, especially if they have substantial behavioral or emotional problems.

Other longer-term residential programs consist of halfway houses and therapeutic communities, also called recovery houses or sober houses. The purpose is generally to allow people to begin the process of reintegration into society while still providing monitoring and support; this is generally believed to reduce the risk of relapse when compared to release directly into society. Postacute residential treatment for adolescents is appropriate for those who are not ready for full reintegration into their homes and communities or whose parents will not allow them to return. Halfway houses are highly variable across programs, including level of therapeutic activities, access to or ability to use psychiatric treatment, supervision, and cost. Therapeutic communities (TCs) are drug-free residential settings that use a hierarchical model with treatment stages that reflect increased levels of personal and social responsibility. Peer influence, mediated through a variety of group processes, is used to help adolescents learn and assimilate social norms and develop more effective social skills. TCs differ from other current treatment approaches principally in their use of the community, comprising treatment staff and others in recovery as key agents of change. In addition to the importance of the community as a primary agent of change, a second fundamental TC principle is "self-help." Self-help implies that the adolescents in treatment are the main contributors to the change process. Mutual self-help means that adolescents also assume partial responsibility for the recovery of their peers, an important aspect of an individual's own treatment. As opposed to halfway houses, there is considerably more evidence for positive treatment outcomes for TCs. Both halfway houses and TCs are almost all 12-step–oriented, using attendance at self-help meetings as a primary therapeutic activity. Although there is modest evidence for the effectiveness of TCs, the variation in the quality of care and specific treatment components suggest that the clinician should take a cautious and considered approach when referring to such programs.

Residential treatment programs such as wilderness therapy, a high-impact, adventure-based therapeutic intervention for adolescents and young adults, are physically and emotionally intense and are based in a wilderness or a remote outdoor setting. Existing research in adventure therapy reports positive outcomes in effectively improving self-concept, self-esteem, help-seeking behavior, increased mutual aid, prosocial behavior, and trust behavior. But there is little evidence (no randomized clinical trials) to support its effectiveness in decreasing substance use.

AFTERCARE

The follow-up for traditional residential treatment approaches has undergone much change over the past several decades. In the past, aftercare might consist of merely sending the adolescent out to attend community

AA or NA meetings, perhaps with a requirement of 90 meetings in 90 days or a similar frequency requirement and with a parent contract requiring strict limits on outside activities and a prohibition of contact with substance-using peers. Progressively, over the last decade or so, formal aftercare groups, individual counseling, and/or family counseling modalities have been established to continue formal treatment after discharge from inpatient or residential treatment.

With limited residential stays, aftercare either in day hospitals, intensive outpatient units, or other outpatient settings has become the site for increasing amounts of adolescent substance abuse treatment. In addition to offering many of the same treatment modalities as inpatient or residential settings, outpatient settings for aftercare often have to concentrate on threats to the adolescent's abstinence. Even for highly motivated youth, the highly protected and structured inpatient setting produces change that cannot be maintained or generalized to the home and the community. More than AA and NA meeting attendance is needed; therefore, aftercare should ideally involve more intensive treatment using behavioral, family modalities and even medication should psychiatric status warrant.

The Adolescent Community Reinforcement Approach

The adolescent community reinforcement approach (A-CRA; Godley et al., 2001) is a behaviorally based intervention that seeks to increase the positive, prosocial day-to-day activities of alcohol and drug-abusing adolescents. The greater access and participation in positive alternative activities the teen has, the fewer opportunities for relapse. A-CRA therapy is accomplished by conducting a functional analysis of using behaviors as well as social activities, developing a list of goals, and monitoring success in these goal areas through personal happiness rating scales. Therapeutic techniques include prosocial and other reinforcer access priming and sampling, problem solving, and communication training. (I describe A-CRA in more detail in Chapter 6.)

Assertive Continuing Care

A-CRA has been adapted for use with assertive continuing care (ACC). ACC uses a combination of case management and A-CRA procedures, including home visits, linking the adolescent to needed services, including existing substance abuse continuing care services. It is a positive (cheerleader) approach with the adolescent and, as previously noted, includes functional analysis of prosocial behavior and explicit procedures to increase prosocial behaviors.

ALTERNATIVE PEER-GROUP PROGRAMS

In the early 1970s, in an effort to deal with increasing drug and alcohol problems among adolescents, the Palmer Methodist Church in Houston, Texas, established a support program providing youth with alternative prosocial activities as a replacement for drug- and alcohol-centered activities, and, in the process, providing an "alternative peer group" for these adolescents. The Palmer Drug Abuse Program (PDAP) is anonymous, free to all adolescents, spiritually based on the 12 steps of Alcoholics Anonymous, and designed to provide social activities in a safe and supportive environment. PDAP has been replicated in at least nine cities in the United States.

In the Houston area, at least six programs describe themselves as "alternative peer-group" (APG) programs, and they are similar to the Palmer program. They have a more expansive menu of therapeutic activities beyond providing prosocial activities. For example, PDAP has expanded its intervention offerings to include crisis intervention, client assessments and referrals, 12-step support group meetings for young people and their parents, individual and family counseling sessions, recovery groups for teens, educational workshops, and supervised weekend retreats and social activities.

The APG model is founded on the assumption that peer relationships, much like the ones that initiate and support drug and alcohol use, are necessary to facilitate recovery (Collier, Hilliker, & Onwuegbuzie, 2014). The goal of this model is to remove the teen from deviant peers and a negatively pressured environment with all its many temptations and triggers and instead offer them a new group of friends that provide positive peer pressure and support for the behavioral changes necessary to promote recovery. Although many of the APG programs have strong 12-step elements, the peer relationship(s) are the focus.

Several factors inherent in the APG model contribute to the recovering adolescent's success. The adolescent is encouraged to learn how to have as much sober fun as possible within healthy boundaries. APGs strive to develop healthy decision making through fun and challenging activities. Parents of teens involved in APGs are encouraged to participate in treatment. Often through parent peer groups, parents examine any behaviors that could possibly be contributing to their adolescent's problems. Parents offer the other parents suggestions on how to change problem behaviors within the family in order to best support their teenager in recovery. Parents may also participate in individual family therapy, which may help teens with any specific issues such as depression or anxiety. APGs work closely with residential treatment programs, psychiatrists, school counselors, and other mental health professionals to provide a more comprehensive, integrated treatment experience. Somewhat similar and often connected to APGs are recovery high schools.

RECOVERY HIGH SCHOOLS

The first wave of recovery high schools opened between 1987 and 1998. Ecole Nouvelle (now Sobriety High) in Minnesota was established in 1986 and opened in a community center with four students and one teacher in 1987. These schools were truly experimental, with the goal of "sober schooling," but they have no existing guidelines or research supporting their effectiveness.

Recovery high schools enroll an average of 30–40 students. The Association of Recovery Schools has about two dozen member high schools. Each school requires students to (1) abstain from substance use and (2) work a program of recovery from substance use (Finch, Tanner-Smith, Hennessy, & Moberg, 2018). Most, though not all, schools are based in the 12-step or Minnesota model of recovery. More than 95% of the students entering recovery high schools have received some form of treatment (residential and/or outpatient services), making recovery schools a source of continuing care support following primary treatment. Unlike treatment facilities, a major focus of recovery schools is education. They are essentially hybrids, serving both continuing care and academic goals. Almost all of the schools have close relationships with extended-care residential treatment programs, halfway houses, and outpatient community treatment programs such as APGs. Most recently, recovery high schools have started to incorporate more treatment programming to address co-occurring mental health disorders.

A more critical issue is consideration of peers in ongoing recovery or aftercare. One of the most salient posttreatment predictors of outcome is participation in prosocial activities. Adolescents who are bright, potentially good students, or have outside prosocial interests such as music, art, or sports have an advantage over most teens who remain peer oriented and often quite resistant to leaving behind even acknowledged deviant peers.

ADEQUATE DURATION OF TREATMENT

Regardless of the level of care or the combination of therapies, adolescents, or for that matter any patient, generally do better with a longer treatment duration. Based on a number of older studies, the concept of 90 days of treatment has been adopted but often expanded to include 90 days of self-help support group attendance (i.e., 90 meetings in 90 days). While it is difficult in these days of managed care to imagine a full 90 days of treatment at more intensive levels of care such as residential, or intensive outpatient, using the 90 days concept as a total across levels seems reasonable. The chronic nature of many SUD cases and psychiatric disorders suggests a long-term approach where monthly or less frequent check-ups might include follow-up assessment for both substance use and associated problems as well as comorbid psychopathology.

If quality programs using evidence-based practices are available, one should reasonably utilize them. As in other areas of behavioral health care, the current community standard is not always based on evidence-based practices but rather on traditional treatments or practices. In the case of adolescent SUD treatment, these are 12-step-based interventions. Although 12-step interventions are not based on a substantial level of scientific evidence but rather on experience gleaned from provider experience, increasing evidence suggests a value for 12-step based facilitation. To a greater or lesser extent, some incorporate elements of evidence-backed practices such as MI, CBT, and family interventions.

TWELVE-STEP INTERVENTIONS

The first and still likely the most widely used approach to the treatment of adolescent substance abuse is an approach based on the philosophy of Alcoholics Anonymous (AA) and Narcotics Anonymous (NA). Treatment programs based on the AA/NA model have been alternatively called self-help programs or Minnesota model programs after the geographical location of the first treatment centers using this model. Despite their ubiquitous use as the basis of treatment programs, they have a limited evidence base. A parallel-group randomized clinical trial comparing 12-step facilitation—which aims to encourage patient participation and engagement in 12-step groups—with MET/CBT in 29 adolescents found no differences in substance use outcomes (Kelly et al., 2017) .

The principles of AA and NA are summarized in the 12 steps that provide a plan for recovery from addiction to alcohol, other drugs, or any one of a number of other "addictions" such as gambling, overeating, or sexual behavior. The AA/NA philosophy is rooted in the belief that change is possible but only if the addicted individual recognizes his or her problem with addiction, admits that he or she cannot control this addiction, and learns to live with it in an adaptive manner. Initial support from a "group" is critical and provides the basis for delivery of the model whether for acute treatment, adjuncts to treatment, or aftercare. Spiritual awareness and growth are seen as critical to the 12-step process.

Later steps promote taking more individual responsibility for one's past behavior and what needs to change in order to achieve a healthier, more adaptive lifestyle and better interpersonal relationships. Acceptance of the disease model of addiction and commitment to an ongoing personal recovery program is useful, if not necessary, for achieving total abstinence from alcohol and other drugs.

Program components of 12-step–based programs include group therapy, lectures, work assignments including 12-step work, a therapeutic milieu, attendance at AA/NA meetings, family therapy or counseling, and recreational activities. Over the past several decades, certified clinicians and other licensed, trained staff have replaced quasi-professional staff at most programs. Ambulatory 12-step programs serve an increasing number of youth compared with past reliance on inpatient, residential programs designed to deliver a basic treatment over 28–42 days. However, managed health care pressures have made residential stays much more variable, depending on individual needs. Many long-term (60 days up to 2 years) programs such as halfway houses and therapeutic communities are also based on AA/NA principles.

Group therapy is the primary mode of treatment delivery within most 12-step programs, although the types and number of group experiences vary among specific programs. In traditional programs, clinicians have relied on psychoeducational groups providing information not only on the adverse effects of drugs and alcohol but also on 12-step principles, personal testimonies about addiction, and ways of dealing with common problems of adolescence. The nonstructured, process-oriented groups have a primary goal of breaking through the denial of group members. Other goals include expressing and clarifying feelings, especially painful affective states, developing relationships, and confronting the negative characteristics or behaviors of adolescents that appear to impede the recovery process. Didactic lectures are often supplemented by videos and audio tapes as well as reading assignments, mostly from the big books of AA/NA.

Another trend within 12-step–based programs involves replacement of the confrontational approach by a more supportive one. A confrontational approach is not useful for most adolescents. Within 12-step–based programs, group therapies are expanding their focus to include cognitive-behavioral methods such as social skills training, which often includes alcohol and other drug refusal skills, problem solving, and relapse prevention. Staff members are also becoming increasingly acquainted with CBT and MI. Many of those with medical staffs are providing assessment and treatment for comorbid psychiatric disorders by providing medications.

Some programs use multifamily groups with staff presenting psychoeducational topics similar to those presented to the adolescents. Additional topics include explaining the process of "enabling" and basic parent management techniques. Multifamily groups also serve an important support function. Families share stories, problems, and advice on adolescent management and problem solving. Parents learn, as do their children, that they are not alone and that others have similar problems. Family programming promotes further parent involvement in such support groups. Family-oriented modalities within AA/NA-based programs attempt to reinforce the idea of the adolescent, and not the parent, taking ultimate responsibility for the adolescent's behavior. Similarly, the adolescent's problem should not be used as an excuse for the parent's behavior, which might include avoidance of marital conflict or job-related problems.

While recovery through the AA and NA 12-step philosophy is described as a lifelong process, completion of the first five steps is considered a satisfactory commitment to abstinence and to continuing the 12-step process after discharge. Individual professionals and treatment programs have developed step workbooks designed specifically for adolescents. Jaffe's (1990) *The Step Workbook for Adolescent Chemical Dependency Recovery* is an example of a simple but complete guide for adolescents to work the first five steps of AA/NA. As in Jaffe's workbook, it is important to explain and work through the 12 steps in a developmentally appropriate fashion. Generally, individual step work is checked and discussed with a clinician on an individual basis and later may be presented to peers in a step study group. Given the reduced time presently allowed during residential stays, the availability of a guide to treatment as well as the importance of outside checks and discussion by both peers and clinicians becomes increasingly important.

Twelve-step programs rely on AA and/or NA to complement treatment and as a major component of aftercare following the completion of acute treatment. The addition of other treatment approaches, including evidence-based interventions, to the core 12-step approach appears to strengthen it. The 12-step approach supplies a useful but not necessary structure for treatment. It offers a method for accepting help and cataloging the adolescent's treatment needs. The availability of support and role models through meetings is an important element in preventing relapse and developing a lifestyle without psychoactive substances.

While this section on 12-step approaches falls in the treatment planning section, I am not advocating 12-step interventions for all adolescents. I do not believe that 12 steps are the only or necessarily the best route to success with adolescents having SUDs. Nevertheless, the potential positives clearly outweigh the negatives at least for 12-step programs incorporating other evidence-based practices. For both adolescents and treatment programs, the identification of AA/NA meetings that are peer-oriented or attended by adequate numbers of adolescents is often useful to the success of recovery and the maintenance of abstinence. Adolescents must feel that meetings are relevant to their concerns. The availability of youthful role models for recovery and the presence of abstinent peers for friendship and support is the actual basis for the self-support movement for adolescents.

GROUP TREATMENT

In SUD treatment programs for adolescents, the most common treatment delivery modality is group therapy in both residential and outpatient care. Group therapy for adolescents has many advantages. It is cost effective, particularly in the context of limited resources such as staff. A number of features associated with group approaches to treatment may facilitate affective, behavioral, and cognitive changes in adolescents with SUDs. These features include the realization that others share similar problems, the development of socializing techniques, role modeling, rehearsal, and peer and therapist feedback. The opportunity to try out new behaviors in a social environment and the development and enhancement of interpersonal learning and trust may also be influential. Because adolescents typically use alcohol or drugs when in the company of their peers, and because they are often easily influenced in group settings, group treatment has the benefit of mirroring their daily experience. Adolescents often prefer groups over other modality options. The social force of cohesiveness (i.e., the degree to which group members are interested in relating to each other) can be used when the group confronts maladaptive and distorted core beliefs. Groups provide a practical forum for such change because of the immediate consensual validation afforded by a group atmosphere.

Earlier claims of iatrogenic effects associated with adolescent group interventions have led to questions about the appropriateness of group-based treatments for substance-abusing youth. Unplanned, incidental interactions among adolescents, referred to as "deviancy training," may be more powerful in influencing an adolescent's future behavior than interactions structured by a group treatment curriculum. More recent studies have largely dispelled this concern, although a variety of other variables need to be considered when assigning adolescents to group, including motivation, level of maturity, severity of deviance and antisocial behavior of the individual members, and the therapist's skill. In other words, group therapy is not for all adolescents. Programs and facilitators are advised to exercise caution when conducting peer groups. Emerging data suggest that this iatrogenic effect may be limited to more deviant, conduct-disordered youth who nevertheless make up a substantial portion of the adolescent SUD treatment population. Other studies show positive effects for group modalities. Clinicians should be cautious when forming groups for treatment and should consider alternative family-based or other modalities for more deviant youths.

I will generally include all adolescents in program group therapies unless they completely refuse, are disruptive in the group setting, or evidence a negative influence on other adolescents in the group. The alternative is a more intensive family or individual therapy approach at least until the adolescent is more receptive to group treatment.

The content of the group therapy delivered is also important. Group interventions based on evidence-based practices such as CBT are preferred and should have treatment manuals as well as therapist training and monitoring procedures. As many evidence-based and nonevidence-based therapies have group formats (e.g., CBT, 12-step groups), the purpose of group therapies is varied. Perhaps the most important purpose of group therapy is to give teens a safe, secure, and self-affirming environment for expression, learning, and recovery. Many programs have generic "process groups" that serve as a support group in which teens speak honestly about their behavior, hold each other accountable for their decisions, and act as positive role models for each other in helping to master the coping skills they need to lead a drug-free life. Particularly in residential programs, process groups are likely to have adolescents at different stages of recovery with varying treatment duration, allowing the more experienced youth to serve as role models for their more novice peers.

There is an ongoing potential for peer groups to deteriorate and adopt a more deviant, resistant tone. Influenced by more negative, deviant peers, adolescents may begin focusing on the perceived positive aspects of their past deviant activities, including substance use, by telling "war stories" and displaying overt oppositional–defiant, resistant behavior to the clinician or program staff. To prevent this resistant behavior from occurring or to deal with it when it does, group clinicians or facilitators need to be vigilant to identify negative, influential peers and assist them in correcting their behavior or remove them from the group.

The Role of Professional Group Facilitators

The role of the support group facilitator should not be to confront the group members or to criticize their behavior. Instead, the therapist's role is to provide structure and to act as a neutral intermediary in guiding the discussion, acting much as a referee at a ball game. The therapist also may serve as an educator, instructing the group on a wide range of topics related to substance abuse and recovery. In the course of a session, a facilitator's role includes:

- Providing structure for the session by enforcing group rules, such as being on time and allowing each member to speak in turn.
- Offering a discussion topic or allowing the group to choose a topic that's relevant to their recovery.

- Fostering participation and positive behaviors such as open, honest communication among group members.
- Discouraging negative behaviors such as extraneous talk, criticism, or confrontational behavior.
- Validating each member's opinions and experiences.
- Identifying group members who may be at risk of a relapse.
- Acting as a role model and advocating for a healthy, drug-free life.

Given the need for skill building in the service of recovery, a relatively unstructured process group may be insufficient by itself to produce lasting change. With changes in group membership and facilitators over time, these groups may be markedly different from one session or program to another. There is no research to establish the efficacy of process groups due primarily to the wide variation in topics discussed and the duration and composition of the group. Nevertheless, they are often part of programs and may offer advantages by increasing engagement and motivation among adolescent group members who feel that their agendas are being considered and discussed. Similarly, group formats for parents and multiple families (including adolescents and parents) for psychoeducation and open process discussion have insufficient data to support their use alone.

For more structured groups such as CBT, the facilitator takes a more active, directive role as per the manual or protocol, but he or she also serves to "direct traffic" in allowing the group to function optimally.

CULTURAL FACTORS

Adolescents in SUD treatment programs come from different backgrounds with various demographic characteristics, including gender, race, ethnicity, physical status, and sexual orientation. These characteristics can affect engagement, motivation, and outcome and therefore should be a concern for the clinician. Clearly, clinicians need not be junior sociologists, but they do need to acknowledge such differences and take steps to address how these differences affect the treatment process.

Race and Ethnicity

An African American or Hispanic working-class adolescent struggling with issues of race, community, economics, and world view may not respond to a particular clinician the same way as a European American from a middle- or upper-middle-class background. Research demonstrates that cultural factors can influence treatment outcome. Adolescents with greater ethnic mistrust (i.e., mistrust of the clinician's different identity) appear to have less response to treatment, and adolescents with greater ethnic pride and ethnic identification demonstrated greater response to treatment. Clinicians need to have a variety of skills in working at multiple levels of influence: individual, microsystems (e.g., family, neighborhoods), and macrosystems (e.g., race and poverty). Cultural, ethnic, and racial differences do not mean that evidence-based interventions do not work for adolescents of a specific background, but aspects of treatment planning and intervention selection may be influenced by the teen's background characteristics. Forcing a particular intervention on adolescents as opposed to allowing some level of choice may serve to reinforce minority adolescents' feelings of subjugation.

Addressing Ethnic and Racial Differences

1. Use of clinicians sharing background characteristics. Youth place greater trust in those from the same ethnic/racial/cultural background and usually assume that the clinician with shared background better understands the adolescent's experience in the world. The use of language or slang used by adolescents from specific groups must be understood and, at least in part, tolerated in order for the clinician to adequately engage adolescents from different cultural backgrounds.

2. Participation of peers sharing background characteristics. Similar to item no. 1, youth feel less alienation if others with their ethnic/racial/cultural background are also participating in treatment. Group treatment is peer treatment, and participants must feel a shared experience with other participants, beyond substance use.

3. Acknowledgment of the reality of the adolescents' daily experience. With all adolescents, clinicians should acknowledge the youths' perceptions of their daily life, including discrimination. Clinicians should demonstrate and understand this experience and how it might affect the adolescent's problems. Assuming this understanding, clinicians can better understand and utilize an appropriate cultural context for the adolescent and his or her family.

4. Emphasis on family interventions, when possible. In many ways, using family interventions avoids the issues of having ethnic/racial/cultural balance in the treatment group. The clinician still has to acknowledge the family's perceptions about their daily experience.

5. Identification of prosocial peer group(s) within the adolescent's environment. Finding appropriate prosocial peer groups must be relevant to the individual adolescent's background and experience. Similarly, the location of such activities needs to be convenient and respect the adolescent's limited economic resources.

Gender

Females are an increasingly larger part of the adolescent SUD treatment population. Female adolescents referred to treatment appear to have more internalizing symptoms and family dysfunction than males. Female adolescent substance users have often experienced severe parental rejection and sexual or physical abuse. They may need more attention to family problems (Kloss, Weller, Chan, & Weller, 2009).

Based on the adult literature, females often present with more problems and tend to function more poorly than males. Male and female adolescents may have different motivations for using drugs, for entering or leaving treatment, and for relapsing. Female and male adolescents influence one another and often distract one another during treatment. Many of the same guidelines for treating adolescents from different ethnic/racial/cultural backgrounds apply to gender. Interventions for adolescents do not have to be segregated. However, if integrated, group interventions need to be reasonably balanced in terms of the backgrounds/identity of both patients and clinicians. Regulating male–female interactions and diverting such interactions from the social to the therapeutic is a challenging aspect of mixed-gender interventions. This challenge can also present an opportunity if clinicians can increase understanding between genders. Interventions addressing internalizing comorbid psychiatric disorders, abuse, and victimization may also need to be a more important part of intervention with female adolescents. Substance use may have an important role in the genesis of female trauma and/or victimization. Substance use may constitute self-medication for trauma-related symptoms; may have facilitated the trauma (e.g., date rape), or both. For some female adolescents, single-gender groups may be necessary to avoid trauma-related sequelae such as flashbacks and to keep them focused on SUD-related topics rather than social interactions and distractions.

Sexual Orientation and Gender Identity

Lesbian, gay, bisexual, and transgender (LGBT) adolescents are at much higher risk for the development of SUDs and other forms of psychopathology than adolescents without these orientations (Marshall et al., 2009). LGBT youth are often struggling with identity issues, are more likely to experience harassment and bullying, and may be subjected to verbal, sexual, and physical abuse and other forms of trauma. The frequent lack of support from parents and other family members makes life and treatment quite challenging for LGBT teens. As a result, they are more likely to drop out of school and even become homeless.

Treatment for SUD among LGBT adolescents may be best provided by organizations specifically serving LGBT teens. These organizations can provide important intervention elements related to the adolescent LGBT experience as well as SUD treatment. Clinicians with LGBT orientation and/or experience can provide an important contribution in adolescent SUD treatment. Unfortunately, such programs and clinicians knowledgeable about LGBT issues are not readily available in all locales. Clinicians need baseline education about the issues confronting LGBT youth and how substance use results and ultimately complicates adjustment. Similar to delivering services to other special populations, clinicians should deliver quality care without bias or prejudice and assist in identifying appropriate services and supports.

Summary of Treatment Planning

Treatment planning for adolescents with SUDs should be determined in part by available resources. Optimally, evidence-based practices provide the foundation for treatment of adolescents with SUDs. Clinicians should consider a combination of modalities to address adolescent motivation and skills deficits, comorbid psychopathology, and impaired family functioning. Targeting identified risk factors for the development and persistence of SUDs provides an excellent framework for treatment planning. While the clinician should preferentially consider evidence-backed practices, nonevidence-based practices such as 12-step–based programs or interventions may be used, especially in concert with evidence-backed practices.

Chapter Six

Cognitive-Behavioral Recovery Skills

Motivation and confidence in one's ability to change are often insufficient to produce persistent improvement in an adolescent's behavior. Many, if not most, adolescents require skills to assist them in behavior change. An essential part of treatment is teaching skills to help adolescents deal with the circumstances that promote and maintain substance use. There are two types of skills: those that specifically deal with substance use and those that deal with deficits commonly associated with substance use problems. Substance use skills include coping with cravings and urges to use substances, managing thoughts about drug use, drug refusal skills, and dealing with lapses and avoiding relapse. Skills for associated deficit include general coping skills, problem-solving skills, anger management, handling of criticism, enhancement of social support networks, and management of negative thinking.

Perhaps the best collection of these skills is CBT, specifically modified for substance use problems. While the classical version of cognitive therapy developed by Aaron Beck addresses the connection between thoughts and feelings, CBT extends this connection to that between thoughts and behavior and is based on a social learning model.

Through a goal-oriented, systematic procedure, CBT aims to solve problems concerning dysfunctional emotions (depression and anxiety), dysfunctional behaviors (substance use and/or other antisocial behaviors), and cognitions (thoughts, feelings, or behaviors). CBT is not a single unitary approach for all behavioral or emotional problems. Rather, it encompasses a number of approaches that vary depending on the treatment components and emphasis. Substantial empirical evidence supports

CBT as being an effective treatment of a variety of problems, including mood, anxiety, personality, eating, substance abuse, and psychotic disorders in children and adolescents (Kendall, 2011). In recent years, CBT models tailored specifically for adolescent substance users have gained significant empirical support. According to the cognitive-behavioral model, adolescents use substances as a maladaptive way of coping with environmental circumstances or getting needs met (Becker & Curry, 2008; Waldron & Kaminer, 2004). Treatment aims to help adolescents replace their drinking or drug use with less risky, prosocial behavior by recognizing the antecedents of their use, avoiding those triggers if possible, and coping more effectively with problems that lead to increased use. Cognitive strategies (e.g., identifying distorted thinking patterns) are typically combined with behavioral strategies (e.g., coping with cravings to use, problem solving, and substance refusal skills). In some models, a motivational enhancement component is offered in the initial sessions. In addition, other skills-focused interventions are often incorporated to promote abstinence, including communication and assertiveness skills, mood regulation through relaxation training, anger management, and modifying cognitive distortions.

The use of modeling, behavior rehearsal, feedback, and homework assignments is characteristic of treatment sessions. Although learning principles would be expected to operate in the same way for adults and adolescents, developmental issues must be addressed to tailor CBT for an adolescent population. Thus, behavioral targets of change (e.g., identification of contingencies) will vary widely depending on the age, developmental level of the adolescent, and his or her specific environmental circumstances. Research findings suggest that the use of substances during the teen years can interfere with crucial developmental tasks, such as prosocial identity formation, acquisition of interpersonal and educational skills, and assumption of family and work responsibilities. Youth who have been heavy users of illicit substances throughout adolescence may not have had sufficient opportunity to acquire certain skills due to preexisting deficits (e.g., ADHD) or the effects of substance use. For such youth, CBT may need to be expanded beyond the topic of substance use to address basic skill deficits, especially problem solving.

KEY COMPONENTS OF CBT FOR ADOLESCENTS WITH SUDs

While specific CBT models vary, most adolescent CBT models for SUDs contain two key components: *functional analysis* and *skills building*. In a functional analysis, the therapist and adolescent(s) work collaboratively to identify the specific thoughts, feelings, events, and circumstances of the adolescent before and after drinking or using drugs. This exercise helps adolescents to identify high-risk situations that lead to increased use while gaining insight into why they drink or use drugs in those situations.

The cognitive-behavioral paradigm assumes that thinking, feeling, and doing are separate realms of the human process that become associated through learning. Substance use, like any behavior, can be linked with thoughts, feelings, and other behaviors through direct experience or through observation. Associations can be strengthened by intense learning experiences or by placement of certain thoughts, feelings, or actions in frequent proximity to use. When they are strong enough, associations can even serve as triggers (i.e., antecedents) that effectively cue or reinforce a person's desire to use—even when that person is planning to abstain. From a cognitive-behavioral perspective, adolescents seeking to change their patterns of cannabis use, for example, should attend to the context in which they use, as well as to the decisions that lead to using. Taking a broad perspective on the context of substance use can improve one's chances for anticipating and thereby avoiding unintended use or ultimately relapse.

Using information obtained through functional analysis, the therapist identifies specific areas where the adolescents would benefit from learning and practicing new skills. Skills that a CBT therapist would commonly consider include assertiveness skills to resist peer pressure, skills for building a social network supportive of recovery, and problem-solving skills for high-risk situations. Commonly used clinician techniques include questioning and testing the adolescent's assumptions about substance use, increasing the teen's pleasant activities, and making assignments for the teen to gradually try out new ways of behaving and reacting.

A Motivational Requirement

Almost all adolescents who use substances receive, or think they receive, some benefit from their substance use. Clinicians must be sensitive to the adolescent's perceptions and not demean them. As noted in Chapter 2, the clinician's role is to assist the teen in assessing these perceived benefits against the risks, impairments, and hassles of use and the benefits of nonuse. Ultimately, at least some of the treatment goals must be endorsed by the adolescent and his or her parents. Some level of motivation is necessary for CBT, although the clinician should be prepared to use MI techniques to resolve lingering resistance and ambivalence about change. In CBT, the emphasis is on skill development and the adolescent's ability to assess assumptions and perceptions about substance use, test these assumptions and perceptions, and develop alternative cognitions and behaviors about use.

Group versus Individual Format

In most studies of CBT for adolescent substance use disorders, CBT has been delivered in a group format. For a program, particularly a residential program or intensive outpatient program, a group format tends to be both feasible and cost effective. However, for the clinician outside a formal program, an individual format is also possible, reasonable, and supported as effective in reducing substance use and related behaviors. Groups have the advantage of adolescents helping their peers and providing meaningful comments, reinforcement, examples of appropriate behavior, and support. In addition to participating in role plays, for example, adolescents can watch their peers perform and participate vicariously. Because such groups are meant to be peer groups, clinicians should have a defined age range (e.g., 13–15 or 16–18 years of age). If co-ed, there should ideally be an adequate number of both genders so that both females and males feel they have peers with whom to identify. Similarly, members of specific ethnic and racial groups should have peers from similar backgrounds. In view of the individual nature of elements of CBT (e.g., specific triggers, maladaptive responses to triggers), the clinician can provide a one- to two-session individual prelude to group CBT in order to conduct a functional analysis for the specific adolescent. Because of the overlap of functional analyses across adolescents, functional analyses can be performed in the group format, with individual adolescents developing the specifics through homework assignments. In the next sections, I discuss the importance and process of a functional analysis, especially the identification of triggers for each adolescent's substance use and skill building. Then I will outline a four-session course of CBT for adolescent SUDs covering the essential topics.

Functional Analysis

A first step in CBT is a functional analysis. The clinician assists the teen in recognizing why he or she is using substances by identifying his or her antecedents for use. This information is then used to determine what the teen needs to do to either avoid or cope with whatever triggers use. This step requires a careful analysis of the circumstances of typical use episodes and the skills and potential resources available to the adolescent. Table 6.1 lists common triggers for substance use. At the conclusion of an initial session of CBT, the clinician should have developed a list of triggers.

The ABC model for understanding and managing behavior is at the core of many effective behavioral strategies (see Figure 6.1). ABC stands for "antecedents," "behavior," and "consequences." "A," antecedents, are what occurs before the behavior—substance use—and include all the relevant things that happened before the behavior occurred. Such precursor behaviors can be considered a trigger for the behavior. "B" is for behavior,

TABLE 6.1. Common Triggers for Substance Use and Relapse

Social

1. Being in the presence of peers or others who use substances.
2. Exposure to places associated with using or being high.
3. Having money.

Interpersonal

1. Conflict with parents, peers, or others.
2. Abuse or neglect.
3. Relationship failure.

Emotional

1. Negative affective states: anger, sadness, loneliness, guilt, fear, and anxiety.
2. Stress.
3. Boredom.
4. Positive affective states: wanting to celebrate.

Life Events

1. Family events: parental conflict, separation, or divorce; departure of a sibling from the home; adolescent leaving home.
2. Social disappointments/separations: breaking up with a boyfriend or girlfriend, feeling rejected by peers, death of a close friend or relative, close friend moving away.
3. Adjustments to new situations: new school, moving away, having legal problems.
4. School- or work-related events: failing in school, getting a new job, losing a job.

which is a description of what happens during the specific behavior, in this case substance use. "C" is for consequences: What are the immediate and delayed results? For substance use, immediate effects include getting high or intoxicated, decrease or increase in dysphoric mood, anxiety, social confidence, problematic sexual situations, fights, and impulsive and illegal behaviors such as stealing. Delayed consequences can include getting into trouble with family, legal problems, health issues, academic difficulties, and vocational problems. The clinician may have obtained information about these domains during the assessment, but a functional

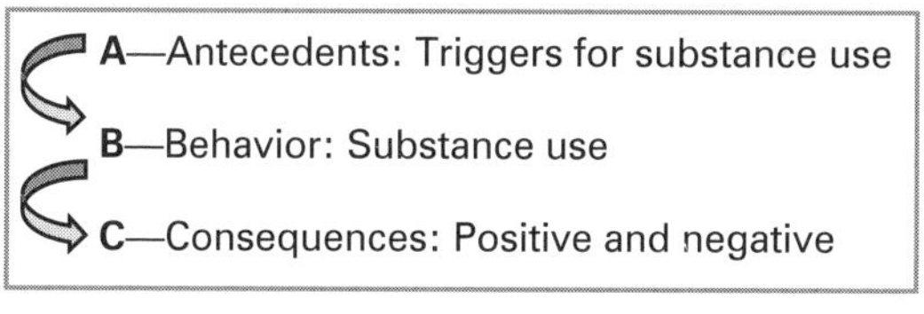

A—Antecedents: Triggers for substance use

B—Behavior: Substance use

C—Consequences: Positive and negative

FIGURE 6.1. The ABC model for understanding behavior.

analysis focuses on specific, usually typical, episodes of substance use rather than a summary of the substance use behavior and consequences. Episodes of nonuse are also valuable for examining how the adolescent responded to triggers without using. The teen can then compare the use and nonuse episodes in terms of the desired outcomes.

The clinician should clarify the determinants and context of substance use obtained from the comprehensive evaluation's questions about the social, environmental, emotional, cognitive, and physical domains. Assuming the functional analysis takes place in an individual session, the clinician can ask the following questions.

Within the *social* domain:

- With whom does the teen spend most of his or her time?
- What is the teen's relationship with others who do not use substances?
- Is the teen living with someone who uses or abuses substances?
- How has the teen's social network changed since he or she started substance use?

Within the *environmental* domain:

- What are specific environmental cues for substance use (e.g., money, alcohol use, times of the day or week, neighborhoods)?
- What is the teen's day-to-day exposure to these cues? Can these cues be avoided (easily)?

Emotional cues include identification of specific negative and positive feelings that commonly precede thinking about or craving substances such as anxiety, depression, anger, boredom, happiness, and excitement.

Cognitive cues involve particular thoughts that precede use.

Physical states such as difficulty concentrating and somatic complaints such as headache, gastrointestinal distress, and withdrawal symptoms may also precede or prompt use.

Clinicians should try to identify the teen's deficiencies and obstacles as well as skills and strengths. The formal functional analysis depends on identifying the determinants of substance use. The determinants for substance use are the triggers for substance use.

Determinants of Substance Use

The clinician can introduce functional analysis to the adolescent as follows: "Triggers are events or activities, persons, and places that often lead to use. Triggers are different for different people. We are going to talk about your triggers."

- What is the adolescent's pattern of use (weekends only, every day, binge use)?
- What triggers his or her substance use?
  - □ Persons (parents, other adults, peers/friends; interactions, conflicts)?
  - □ Places (school, home, friends, parks, etc.)?
  - □ Things (events, memories, mood, or other emotional states)?

CLINICIAN: Are there any particular places where you use?

ADOLESCENT: At friends' homes, in cars; sometimes, but rarely, at my house.

CLINICIAN: Specific people with whom you are more likely to use?

ADOLESCENT: My boyfriend, now; with my friend Suzie . . . and their friends.

CLINICIAN: Do all your friends trigger thoughts about using or using itself?

ADOLESCENT: No, I have a few nonusing friends.

CLINICIAN: What is the difference between using and nonusing friends?

ADOLESCENT: I think my using friends are screw-ups like me.

CLINICIAN: Are there feelings or situations that are more likely to lead to your using? For example, feeling sad, mad, or bored?

ADOLESCENT: Mostly bored. I am really not much into school. Even when I am with my friends, it often gets boring. Of course, when I am upset, I like to use.

CLINICIAN: Does thinking about certain things, such as certain memories of past events, make you want to use?

ADOLESCENT: I guess I want to use when I think about how screwed up my life is now. I feel like a failure. I often think about my old boyfriend who broke up with me—he said I used too much.

CLINICIAN: So feeling bad about the consequences of your use—trouble, loss of relationships—makes you want to use even more? [reflection, an MI technique. MI can be used throughout CBT or other interactions to facilitate an adolescent's desire to change.]

- Does the adolescent use substances alone or with other people? Is either a trigger?
- Where does the teen buy and use substances? Are they given to the adolescent by specific others (girl/boyfriend, sibling, parent, other adult, or friend)?
- Where and how does the adolescent get the money to buy drugs?
  - □ Allowance?
  - □ Stealing or other illegal behavior?
  - □ Gift(s)?
- What has happened to the teen before the most recent episodes of use?
  - □ Events (conflicts, trauma including abuse and/or neglect)?
  - □ Memories of events?

CLINICIAN: Let's think about the last several times you used. What was happening right before you decided to use? How long before you actually used after you decided to use?

ADOLESCENT: Oh, I knew I was going to an evaluation and probably then to rehab. So I was mad at my parents and upset at myself. I had to use one more time, so I went outside to the backyard.

CLINICIAN: How did that work?

ADOLESCENT: I felt much better . . . for a while. It made me tired and I got to sleep. But in the morning . . . nothing had changed—I was still going to rehab.

- What circumstances were at play when substance use began or became a problem?
- How does the teen describe substances and their effects?
- What are the roles, both positive and negative, that substance use plays in the teen's life?

CLINICIAN: Have there been times when you had decided *not* to use but encountered a trigger that prompted or drove you to use?

ADOLESCENT: Sometimes it's hard. But usually there is something else to do or to distract me—or I hang out with a nonusing friend.

For the teen in the preceding dialogues, the primary triggers are (1) boredom, (2) intense emotion, (3) certain friends who also use, and (4) places where she had commonly used. In addition to broad categories of use, the clinician should also list specific examples under each category, for example, particular emotions and specific instances, all using friends, and the specific places where the adolescent commonly uses.

Perhaps the cornerstone of CBT is the trigger list for each teen. The adolescent needs to master this list and be able to anticipate when these triggers might occur and in what situations.

Skills Building

The other part of CBT is the development of skills to deal with triggers. Toward this end, the skills-building part of CBT is delivered with two broad treatment objectives in mind: (1) teach adolescents how to anticipate and challenge triggers—the thoughts, cravings, and urges that drive substance use—and (2) teach adolescents how to use a broader range of adaptive responses, skills, or coping activities to help deal with or avoid the triggers. Substance use can be seen as a maladaptive form of coping. Developing adaptive coping skills will have the effect of reducing the need for alcohol or other drugs as coping agents. Similarly, by reducing or eliminating substance use, adolescents learn alternative approaches to problem solving, coping, and stress management that have greater potential for long-term benefit and improved functioning.

The core skills taught in a four-session version of CBT for adolescents with SUDs are problem solving, managing thoughts about alcohol and drugs, coping with cravings, and planning for lapses. These core topics, discussed in the rest of this chapter, are directly related to substance use. Other possible skills are commonly associated with use, particularly for adolescents, such as anger control, communicating with parents, and coping with psychiatric comorbidity such as depression. Skills are taught through a combination of clinician modeling and adolescent role plays, as described in detail later in this chapter, along with assigned homework practice (see Figure 6.2).

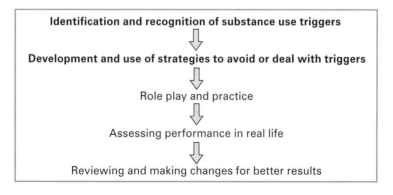

FIGURE 6.2. Sequence of CBT for SUDs.

CBT FOR ADOLESCENTS WITH SUDs

The rest of this chapter describes a four-session course of group CBT for adolescents with SUDs. Sessions can be scheduled weekly or even twice a week, last between 60 and 75 minutes, and ideally have between six and eight adolescents per group in order to maximize individual adolescent participation. There are pros and cons to coed groups. Opposite-sex members are often distracting and may prompt theatrics to impress. However, the presence of members of the opposite sex may serve to make their opposite-sex peers be more honest by calling them on their more outrageous statements. Regardless, if the group is coed, there should be a reasonable balance of males and females. Because of potential developmentally based cognitive differences, groups should be separated into a younger group (<14 years) and an older group (15–18 years), within which there can be differences in severity of use and comorbidities. There can be one or two group leaders, at least one of whom should have experience with this patient population. Inappropriate group members are usually those with high social deviance and poor motivation. This type of patient may persist at trying to negatively influence peers and generally disrupt the group. If group dynamics and clinician skills are unable to mitigate their negative influence or disruptive behavior, these adolescents should be excused from the group.

Clinician Skills and Roles

Training in CBT is critical for optimal administration of this form of recovery skills therapy. Knowledge of the concepts supporting CBT will allow the clinician to reach across commonly associated areas of dysfunction such as substance use *and* depression *and* anxiety *and* anger control. Considering the range of problems present in the "average" adolescent with SUDs, the more skills that can be taught within a single CBT treatment course, the more efficient and potentially effective the intervention becomes in improving the adolescent's overall functioning.

In the group CBT format, the clinician follows the outline for a specific session of CBT but allows the adolescent group members to do as much work as possible by reviewing their homework, assisting peers by prompting responses, and role playing. The value of the group approach is the interaction it allows between peers, spreading participation around so it is not dependent on one or two adolescents and thereby enabling teens to learn from a variety of their peers. Learning can be improved through clinician modeling and adolescent role playing to engage adolescents in the group exercises. Adolescents then role-play scenes based on personal experience to help ground the skill in real-life events.

It's also important to acquaint parents with the skills that are being taught so that they can reinforce them. Parents may notice improved overall problem solving, anger control, and ability to access a prosocial peer group. Acknowledging these efforts may reinforce positive adolescent progress in recovery. In addition, the adolescent often needs to be prepared for working with his or her parents on communication and family problem-solving skills.

Session Topics and Session Structure

The CBT session core topics are listed in Table 6.2. The order of presentation of topics deserves discussion, as the various examples of CBT often differ in the way they order these skills. The amount of time available for treatment often dictates this ordering, as one must deal directly with substance topics before general topics. Acquisition of CBT and SUD skills often involves problem solving, essentially the problem(s) caused by the presence of a trigger and the adolescent's ability to deal with the trigger in an adaptive manner. However, problem-solving skills can be a useful lead-in to nonsubstance-related topics when time allows. I advocate dealing initially with the identification of triggers in Session 1; next, problem solving in Session 2; and finally, as a basis for discussion of SUD topics, Sessions 3 and 4. Then, if needed and as time allows, one can present some of the general functioning topics, such as dealing with depression, anxiety, or other aversive mood states; anger control; and conflict management.

Each of the sessions follows a typical sequence:

1. Review of client status.
   - Substance use.
   - Use of skills.
2. Review of practice (homework).
3. Introduction of new skill/rationale for use.
4. Skill-use guidelines: modeling and role playing.
5. Group exercise.
6. Homework and real-life practice exercises.

TABLE 6.2. Introduction to Communication Skills: Core Session Topics for CBT for Adolescent SUDs

1. Identifying triggers (functional analysis).
2. Problem solving.
3. Managing thoughts about drugs/alcohol; coping with cravings and urges to use.
4. Crisis control: Planning for lapses and other emergencies.

Despite the structured nature of CBT, it is essential to recognize the adolescent's real-life and often more acute problems. Each session should begin with a 10-minute review of the client's current status, that is, what has been happening since the last session. This component provides a brief period of supportive therapy for adolescents to discuss their current problems related to substance use or abstinence. It also provides the clinician and other group members with the opportunity to support adolescents who are having difficulty and to congratulate those who are achieving success. The individual problems of the group are grist for the mill and can be used as examples of triggers and problems to be solved using their new cognitive skills.

Session 1: Identifying Triggers (Functional Analysis)

Session Outline

- Introductions, treatment overview, group rules, homework.
- Introducing the ABC model of substance use.
- Skill-use guidelines: modeling and role playing.
- Group exercises.
  - □ Exercise 1: Make a list of triggers.
  - □ Exercise 2: Map the ABCs of use.
- Homework and real-life practice exercises.
  - □ Review and add to trigger list.
  - □ If triggers occur between sessions, log what you did in response to it.

Materials Needed

- Handout: Functional analysis worksheet (Figure 6.3).

Introductions, Treatment Overview, Group Rules, Homework

In the first session, adolescents will not have homework to review. Instead, the clinician provides an overview of CBT and the topics to be covered. The clinician also explains the importance of homework and practice to master skills. The clinician then reviews group rules (attendance; expectations for participation, behavior; confidentiality). The adolescents should introduce themselves and be asked to answer a benign question such as, "What would people be surprised to know about me?" The clinician can then ask adolescents to state their expectations for the group.

Introducing the ABC Model of Substance Use

The clinician presents the ABC model of substance use behavior and the importance of knowing what prompts substance use, what keeps it going, and its consequences—positive and negative, short-term and long-term.

"Triggers are events, activities, persons, and places that often lead to use. Examples include going out with certain friends, going to places such as parties or concerts, or riding in cars around town. Triggers also include feelings or emotions that you have such as feeling sad, angry, or anxious. And sometimes they involve both people and feelings—seeing someone from a failed relationship and becoming sad or upset or becoming angry when you are with your parents, with whom you may have conflicts. Triggers are different for different people. We are going to talk about your triggers."

The clinician defines external triggers, internal triggers, specific substance use behavior, and consequences (short-term positive effects and short- and long-term negative consequences). Also, the clinician discusses what adolescents expect to happen when they use specific substances—for example, changes in mood and feelings, escape from feelings or circumstances, changes in perception, increased enjoyment of activities, greater social ability and attractiveness. Ask:

"Do these expectations come true?"
"How do these consequences from substance use fit with your goals for your life?"

Skill-Use Guidelines: Modeling and Role Playing

The clinician provides examples of using the ABC paradigm, giving several examples of specific triggers and consequences of hypothetical substance use, asking for adolescent comment throughout.

In group settings, the clinician may want to make modeling and role playing as fun-filled and entertaining as possible, playing ineffective (e.g., passive, aggressive, passive–aggressive) and effective (assertive) responses to specific triggers or situations.

Group Exercises

EXERCISE 1: MAKE A LIST OF TRIGGERS

Divide space on a blackboard or whiteboard into external triggers (people, places, and things) and internal triggers (feelings). After each trigger is endorsed and placed on the board in the front of the room, ask group members to raise their hands if the trigger applies to them. If so, have them list the trigger on a piece of paper or device that they are to maintain. Always elicit comments about the exercise and the responses from the adolescents.

EXERCISE 2: MAPPING THE ABC'S OF USE

Using detailed examples from their recent experience(s), have one to two adolescents identify the specific ABC's. For example, the teen would say: "This specific trigger occurred, I used this substance in the following pattern, resulting in these positive consequences and these negative consequences [if any consequences]." For example:

> "I went out riding with some of my using friends. No one wanted to go anyplace in particular; we got bored and stopped in a parking lot and lit up some joints. We got high. I got home late—I lost track of time. I also forgot that I had to show up at the magistrate's office on Monday and that I might have a pee test, which now was definitely going to be positive."

Provide the adolescent with Figure 6.3.

Homework and Real-Life Practice Exercises

Teens are to review their trigger lists and add any additional triggers. If any triggers occur between the sessions, they are to log what they did in response to the trigger.

Session 2: Problem Solving

Clinicians may elect to place the session on problem solving first or even later in the order of sessions. Introduce the problem-solving paradigm to assist adolescents in working through decisions they will have to make when confronted by triggers or other high-risk situations. The use of a single, simple paradigm allows adolescents to develop a meta-skill that can serve them in a variety of problem areas.

One potential problem with approaches based on problem solving is the common occurrence of impulsivity or emotionally driven behaviors in adolescents with SUDs. The immediacy of the trigger, concurrent affective symptoms, the high level of salience of the trigger, as well as adolescent impulsivity, might prevent the adolescent from using the steps—or using them successfully. It is important that the adolescent be involved in

Preparing to Conduct a Functional Analysis: Identifying Your Triggers

This worksheet will help you to identify the circumstances, situations, people, locations, thoughts, and feelings that increase the likelihood that you will use stimulants.

- List the places where you frequently used stimulants.
- List the people with whom you frequently used or purchased stimulants.
- List the times or days when you most frequently used stimulants.
- List the kinds of activities in which you were typically engaged when you used stimulants.
- List the feelings and emotions that you experienced after you were exposed to triggers.
- List the kinds of things that you were thinking about after you were exposed to triggers.

Trigger	Feelings and Thoughts	Your Behavior	Positive Consequences	Negative Consequences

(continued)

FIGURE 6.3. Functional analysis worksheet.

Conducting a Functional Analysis of Your Substance Use

Step 1:

In the column titled "Your Behavior," briefly describe an example in which you recently used substances.

Step 2:

Think about what you were doing immediately prior to this episode of substance use. Can you remember who you were with, what you were doing, or the time of day? Place these in the "Trigger" column.

Step 3:

Immediately prior to using substances during this episode, what were you thinking about? Do you remember what you were feeling? Place whatever thoughts and feelings that you can remember in the "Feelings and Thoughts" column.

Step 4:

What happened immediately after you used the substances? How did your mood change? Did you feel euphoric or powerful? Did you feel that you had more energy or power than normal? Did you feel happy or not as depressed as before? Did you stop feeling bad about something?

Step 5:

What have been the long-term consequences of this and other episodes of substance use? How has it affected your relationships with friends? How has it affected your family? How has it affected your work or school situation? How has it affected your financial situation? How has it affected your emotional health? How has it affected your physical health?

Return to Step 1:

Describe another example of a relatively recent episode of substance use. Repeat all the steps as before. Repeat this until the worksheet has been completely filled.

FIGURE 6.3. *(continued)*

looking at alternative behaviors and choosing an adaptive response(s). In other words, having considered triggers and possible responses, the adolescent needs to arrive at a specific adaptive response that he or she agrees to use whenever the trigger is encountered. Experience tells us that in the heat of the moment, adolescents will be unable to systematically go through the "steps" and think about problem solving. I suggest an emphasis on identifying a list of prominent triggers and running through the steps with repeated practice in order to establish *scripts* that can become automatic, adaptive responses. This requires an emphasis on identifying and anticipating triggers, especially in the context of certain persons (parents, peers), places (school, home), and "things" (emotions, thoughts) and having the adaptive response come immediately due to prior consideration and practice.

Session Outline

- Review of client status.
- Review of practical homework.
- Introduction of problem solving and its rationale.
  - Step 1: Recognize that a problem exists and identify the problem or trigger.
  - Step 2: Come up with possible solutions to the problem or responses to the trigger.
  - Step 3: Evaluate possible solutions and choose one.
  - Step 4: Try the chosen solution and evaluate how it turned out.
- Skill-use guidelines: Modeling and role playing.
- Group exercise: Adolescents are to generate problem situations and work through the steps.
- Homework and real-life practical exercises.
  - Take a problem that arises and go through the problem-solving steps, writing them down.
  - Continue to keep a trigger log.

Materials Needed

- Blackboard, whiteboard, or posterboard and marker.
- Handout: Problem-solving steps (Figure 6.4).

Review of Client Status

At the beginning of this and each subsequent session, the clinician asks the group for any updates on their general functioning and activities since the last session. The clinician may also go around the room and query each teen for an update, accepting that some adolescents may be reluctant to talk or provide information. The adolescents are encouraged to provide information about their substance use, particularly as it relates to triggers and consequences. In subsequent sessions, the clinician should query teens about their use of CBT skills taught in previous sessions.

Review of Practice Homework

Homework assignments are reviewed by asking for volunteers and calling on specific teens. The clinician should provide encouragement for participation and positive reinforcement when active participation occurs but should not punish nonparticipation. The clinician should attempt to ignore occasional irrelevant or negative comments from the group members, actively intervening only if the comments persist or have an obvious influence on group behavior.

Introducing Problem Solving and Its Rationale

> "Adolescents run into all sorts of difficult situations that require decisions, such as whether to use drugs or alcohol, go to school, stay out all night without permission, smoke cigarettes, have sex, and get into physical fights or arguments. Even more often, teenagers have less serious decisions to make such as whether to do homework or do one's household chores. Of course, decisions have consequences. Good decisions may result in a pat on the back, getting an allowance, and gaining extra privileges. Bad decisions often result in negative consequences such as bad grades, losing an important relationship, being grounded, or losing privileges such as video game time, cell phone use, or use of the car. Even more serious consequences are having to go to rehab or undergo some type of treatment."

The clinician should ask for examples of recent problems and resulting decisions and consequences.

> "Triggers are a kind of problem situation where a decision has to be made. In order to make better decisions, we have problem-solving steps."

The steps of the problem-solving model include the following.

STEP 1: RECOGNIZE THAT A PROBLEM EXISTS AND IDENTIFY THE PROBLEM OR TRIGGER—"IS THERE A PROBLEM AND WHAT IS IT?" OR "IS A TRIGGER PRESENT OR ANTICIPATED?"

Individually, each adolescent has been asked to develop a list of triggers and should be prepared to discuss them in the group setting. The adolescents should be able to help the group construct a master list of triggers for the group, reinforcing the common occurrence of most of the triggers across the group of teens. Problem or trigger recognition is perhaps the most important single skill in CBT. The clinician can introduce an exercise on triggers as follows:

"From our discussion of what happened to each of you since our last session, let's identify the triggers that the group encountered."

Discussion of trigger recognition and exposure (during the period since the last session) should be part of every session.

STEP 2: COME UP WITH POSSIBLE SOLUTIONS TO THE PROBLEM (OR RESPONSES TO THE TRIGGER)—"WHAT CAN I DO?"

Brainstorm with the group members to think of as many solutions as you can. Think of solutions that involve thoughts and behavior. Include solutions or responses that group members have made in the past and ones that they should make (i.e., more adaptive responses). Coming up with bad solutions is useful to provide a bit of humor and fun and also to emphasize that bad decisions are often made.

> CLINICIAN: Let's think of *every* possible response to the problem of having your best friend ask you to skip class and go smoke some reefer.
>
> ADOLESCENT 1: You could say, "No, I have to go to class or I'll fail this quarter."
>
> CLINICIAN: OK, what about another response?
>
> ADOLESCENT 2: Sure, let's go . . . as long as it's good stuff.
>
> CLINICIAN: Yes, that is a possible response. Any other possible responses?
>
> ADOLESCENT 3: You could just say maybe later . . . just to get the friend off your back.

STEP 3: EVALUATE POSSIBLE SOLUTIONS AND CHOOSE ONE—
"WHAT WILL HAPPEN IF . . . ?"

Before action, teens should consider all the positive and negative short- and long-term consequences of each alternative, even the bad ones. Each teen should choose one option that is likely to solve the problem with the least amount of hassle or trouble to him or her and others. Positive consequences should be reinforced and praised, while negative consequences should be discussed among the group members to be certain they agree that the consequences are indeed negative.

> CLINICIAN: The group has provided several options. Let's consider the likely result if you did each of these.
>
> ADOLESCENT 1: If I said no, my friends would probably bother me until I went with them.
>
> ADOLESCENT 2: If I went and smoked, I might get into trouble from skipping or might be caught using.
>
> ADOLESCENT 3: If I said later, my best friend would probably forget about it. . . .

STEP 4: TRY THE CHOSEN SOLUTION AND EVALUATE HOW IT TURNED OUT—
"HOW DID IT WORK?"

After each teen has tried the solution, ask "Does it seem to be working? If not, consider what you can do to make the plan work, or give it up and try the next best solution." This step is critical in review of homework and the group members' actual experience(s).

> CLINICIAN: I know that Billy and Joanne each reported several offers to use since our last session. How did it go?
>
> BILLY: My best friend kept at it until I went with him, skipped my last class, and shared a joint with him. I just found out that I missed too many classes, and I have to go to summer school or flunk. Of course, I was also positive on my pee test.
>
> JOANNE: I told Susie—maybe later. . . . She got caught using and is going to court.

Group members should work on the problem recognition stage, with particular emphasis on describing the problem in as much detail as possible. The group can brainstorm, coming up with alternative choices and writing them on the blackboard or posterboard. Have the group reason through the process of weighing alternatives, looking at both positive and negative and short- and long-term consequences. The group should prioritize the alternatives and then choose one. Either put this solution on hold and go through the model again with another problem or elicit volunteers and begin role playing.

Skill-Use Guidelines: Modeling and Role Playing

See the above examples. Demonstrate an example from elicited problems and proceed through the steps.

Group Exercise

Obtain problem examples from adolescents and have individual adolescents work through steps, getting help as needed from peers.

To encourage role playing among group members, clinicians should start by having them generate problem situations of mild to moderate difficulty and only later have them move to more difficult situations. Clinicians can use the following strategies to help adolescents generate problem situations:

- Ask adolescents to recall a recent problem situation in which another solution would have been desirable.
  "I was afraid to speak up when one of my teachers asked a question in class. . . . I knew the answer."
  "I screamed at my mom when I could have asked nicely . . . she might have let me go with my friend to the mall."
- Ask adolescents to anticipate a difficult situation that may arise in the near future in which problem solving could be used.
  "My little sister is always borrowing my clothes. . . . I want to ask her to stop, but I usually just yell and scream."
- Suggest an appropriate situation based on knowledge of a participant's recent circumstances.
  "John, you told the group that you are missing school after using a lot at night due to marijuana use after fighting with your parents. Is that a trigger for use?"
- Help adolescents generate details about a given situation by identifying its location, the key figures involved, and the essential problem or trigger being faced. In role-play and group exercises in general, the key to successful teaching is processing what actually occurs.

CLINICIAN: Tracey, when you came in this afternoon, you mentioned that you had a bad day yesterday. Can you share what happened?

ADOLESCENT: I had a fight with my boyfriend.

CLINICIAN: Let's try to identify the trigger. Where were you, and what was happening before you had the fight? What were you doing? What do you think caused the fight?

Participation in an exercise or role play should always be met with the clinician's praise or recognition for practice and improvement. Constructive criticism about the less effective elements of the adolescents' behavior is always easier for clients to take once they have been told that their participation is appreciated and they've been informed about any positive aspects of their responses. Peer comments are also useful and allow the group to develop improved communication skills in providing constructive comments—both positive and negative.

Homework and Real-Life Practice Exercises

- Handout: Problem-solving steps (Figure 6.4).
- Practice exercise: Adolescents are to take the problem that arises in the interim period and go through the problem-solving steps, ideally writing down each step alternative and response.
- Continue to maintain the trigger log.

Session 3: Coping Skills for Cravings to Use Substances, Including Refusal Skills

This set of skills is synonymous with managing thoughts about substance use. With the addition of refusal skills, the clinician is dealing with a specific problem or behavior.

Step 1: Recognize that a problem exists and identify the problem or trigger.
Step 2: Come up with possible solutions to the problem (or responses to the trigger).
Step 3: Evaluate possible solutions and choose one.
Step 4: Try the chosen solution and evaluate how it turned out.

FIGURE 6.4. Problem-solving steps.

Session Outline

- Review of client status.
- Review of practice homework.
- Introduction of coping skills for cravings and thoughts about substance use.
  - □ Managing urges and cravings.
  - □ Managing thoughts about alcohol and drugs.
    - Challenge thoughts about substance use.
    - List and recall the benefits of not using.
    - List and recall unpleasant drinking and drug experiences.
    - Use distractions.
    - Self-reinforcement.
    - Decide to delay.
    - Leave the situation or change it.
    - Call for support.
  - □ Refusal skills.
  - □ Skill-use guidelines—Modeling and role playing.
    - Demonstration Exercise 1: Clinician demonstrates use of several techniques for coping with cravings and urges.
    - Demonstration Exercise 2: Adolescents offer clinician drugs or alcohol, and the clinician demonstrates refusal responses.
    - Teen Group Exercise 1: The first two teens start as the friend and the subject, respectively. The friend offers the subject an opportunity to use and the subject responds. Once this interaction has run its course, the subject becomes the friend and so on until each adolescent has had a chance to be both the friend and the subject. The clinician debriefs the group on the exercise and which subject responses would be most effective in the real world.
    - Teen Group Exercise 2: The clinician makes offers "to use" to each adolescent, who then replies with a drug refusal statement. After each adolescent has a chance to respond to the clinician's offers, the group is debriefed.
- Homework
  - □ Develop a personalized craving plan.
  - □ Review triggers list.
  - □ Keep a craving/urges log along with a triggers log.

Materials Needed

- Blackboard, whiteboard, or posterboard and marker.

Review of Client Status

Review activities and general functioning, substance use triggers encountered and adolescents' responses, and their use of problem-solving skills.

Review of Practice Homework

Review problem-solving steps (see if adolescents can recall the steps without a visual aid) and trigger logs.

Go over several of the adolescents' problems and their problem-solving steps.

Introducing Coping Skills for Cravings and Thoughts about Substance Use

MANAGING URGES AND CRAVINGS

Begin by again emphasizing the importance of identifying and anticipating triggers so that adolescents can develop plans to respond, including reducing their exposure to these triggers. Explain that there are not only physical triggers (people and places) but also physical symptoms (jitter, tightness in stomach), cognitive signs (increased thoughts, usually positive, about use and preoccupation with use) and psychological signs (depression, anxiety). These triggers commonly produce cravings, which are best described as increasing thoughts, and ultimately preoccupation with use.

> "Craving is a trigger. Craving is most often experienced early in treatment or abstinence, but episodes of craving may persist—at least intermittently—for weeks, months, and sometimes even years after you stop drinking or using drugs. Craving may be uncomfortable, but it is a very common experience. You should expect craving to occur, and so you should be prepared to cope with it if and when it occurs. Though of variable duration, craving and urges are time-limited; that is, they usually last only a few minutes and at most a few hours. Rather than increasing steadily until they become unbearable, cravings usually peak after a few minutes and then die down, like a wave. Urges will become less frequent and less intense as you learn how to cope with them."

Beyond learning to identify and reduce exposure to triggers, coping with urges or craving (to use) includes involvement in distracting activities, talking with supportive family and friends, or attending self-help support groups. "Urge surfing" is another skill similar to relaxation training or to mindfulness as practiced in dialectical behavioral therapy (DBT).

"Some urges, especially in the early stages of recovery, are just too strong to ignore. When this happens, it can be useful to stay with urges or cravings to use until they pass. Urges are a lot like ocean waves. They are small when they start, grow in size, and then break up and dissipate. You can imagine yourself as a surfer riding the wave, staying on top of it until it crests, breaks, and turns into harmless, foamy surf.

"When experiencing a craving, many people have a tendency to remember only the positive effects of alcohol or drugs and often forget the negative consequences. Therefore, when experiencing craving, it can be helpful to remind yourself of the negative consequences of substance use as well as the benefits of abstinence. Sometimes it is helpful to have these benefits and consequences listed on a small card or on your smartphone that you can keep with you. Developing positive or adaptive self-talk can assist with this process. What you tell yourself about your urges to drink will affect how you experience and handle them. Self-talk can be put to use to strengthen or weaken urges and cravings."

Consistent with cognitive therapy techniques is learning to challenge and modify one's thoughts about substance use. In time, the process of making positive self-statements can become automatic; it is much more adaptive than negative self-talk or statements. So group members need to practice, practice, practice. The group setting allows peers to provide examples of self-talk in order to prompt or remind one another of potential examples.

MANAGING THOUGHTS ABOUT ALCOHOL AND DRUGS

Not all thoughts about drugs and alcohol immediately trigger urges or cravings to use, although thoughts have the potential to do so. Thinking about alcohol and/or drugs is not necessarily a problem as long as one doesn't *act* on those thoughts. Some adolescents may feel guilty about the thoughts (even though they have not acted on them), and they may try to get them out of their minds. An important CBT skill is learning to identify those thoughts or feelings that can lead to drinking or drugging and then learn some new ways to catch themselves before an actual slip or lapse. These thoughts are among the triggers to be identified. Recovering adolescents need to be aware of states of mind (e.g., anxiety, depression, loneliness, anger) that can predispose them to use or ultimately to relapse. It is not the thinking itself that creates the problem but how teens deal with it. Substance users can learn to dismiss this thinking from their minds whenever it appears, recognize it for what it is, or counter it with contrary thoughts; it need not lead to a relapse. Although many of the triggers for urges and cravings are the same for thoughts about substance use, other triggers include nostalgia for use, testing one's control (after a period of sobriety), a crisis, adverse mood states, self-doubts, escape from unpleasant situations (e.g., disappointment, failure embarrassment), wanting to relax, negative self image, and interpersonal difficulties (conflict, failed or problem romance). Particularly for adolescents, socialization with peers is paramount. Many adolescents who are shy or very uncomfortable in social situations feel the need for a social lubricant. CBT suggests several techniques for dealing with such problem thoughts.

Challenging Thoughts. Use other thoughts to challenge the resumption thoughts. An important aspect of challenging thoughts is do *not* visualize what one is *not* going to do; picture a substitute or opposing behavior that one *is* going to do. To begin a new habit, adolescents should have a behavioral image of themselves engaging in the new behavior, not just on occasion but every time the unwanted habit pops into mind.

List and Recall the Benefits of Not Using. Thoughts about the personal benefits of abstinence can help weaken your excuses for drinking. Benefits to think about include staying out of trouble, not disappointing friends and relatives, increased self-esteem, and sense of self-control. It is important to pay attention to these positive aspects of abstinence and to the progress you are making, rather than focusing on what you seem to be giving up. Add more items of your own to the list of benefits. Carry a card listing the benefits of abstinence, which you should review whenever you catch yourself being persuaded to use drugs or alcohol.

List and Recall Unpleasant Drinking and Drug Experiences. Try to recall the pain, fear, embarrassment, and other negative feelings associated with drinking. Make a list of the unpleasant experiences associated with substance abuse, such as blackouts, hangovers, fist fights, arrests, and withdrawal. Try to conjure up an *image* of a specific unpleasant experience. Make a list of the negative effects of drinking on the reverse side of the card listing the benefits of sobriety. At moments of temptation, take out the card and read it over slowly three or four times. One needs to counteract the "pros" of substance abuse with the "cons" of substance use and the "pros" of sobriety. Think beyond the immediate pleasure associated with alcohol or drugs, playing out the mental image of a using episode to its conclusion; include all the negative consequences that could arise if substance use occurs.

Use Distractions. Develop a list of distracting thoughts, ideas, and activities. Thinking about something unrelated to substance use can stop thoughts about it. For example, think about pleasant, enjoyable topics such as prosocial weekend plans, family members, relaxation, and favorite hobbies or activities. Focusing on a task you want to complete is another constructive distraction. As the adolescent develops more prosocial activities and interests, these should be added to the list of possible distracting thoughts.

Self-Reinforcement. Teens need to remind themselves of their recovery success so far, for example, 3 weeks of abstinence, becoming actively involved in treatment, staying in the treatment program, working harder, and making improved grades at school.

Decision Delay. Put off any decision to use drugs or alcohol for 15–30 minutes. Most urges to use drugs are like waves; they build to a peak and then diminish, at which time they may be more manageable or pass altogether. If you wait a while, the wave will pass. Imagine that you are a surfer riding the "wave" of craving until it subsides, or use another image that is effective for you.

Leave the Situation or Change the Situation. Leave or change the situation in which you start having thoughts about using drugs. Adolescents should have a list of alternative activities or physical exercise ready.

Call for Support. Call someone—a sponsor, friend, or family member—who in the past has been helpful talking you through a high-risk situation.

Refusal Skills

Abstinence or decreased substance use often hangs on adolescents' ability to handle peer requests to use or to avoid peer behavior that would expose them to triggers to use. Such peer requests and pressure may be overt or subtle; they may not involve an invitation to use but will expose the teen to triggers. Overcoming peer pressure, whether perceived or overt, is among the hardest tasks for adolescents in recovery. Discussion in a group setting of adolescents with similar problems reminds each member of the group's empathy and understanding of the difficulty of saying "no." However, "no" is not the only possible response, and the group can present a number of response options that preserve perceived peer social standing.

> "Friends are going to ask you to use. This might happen in a setting where it is easy to decline. Often, asking to use may occur in the presence of other triggers and peer pressure to use. You have to be prepared with strategies and statements to use in order to refuse to use."

Adolescents need to prepare to be asked to use just as they need to prepare for other triggers. They should be ready with at least several strategies when asked. Rehearsal of these responses is critical, as teens should speak clearly and firmly with direct eye contact.

"While an emphatic 'no' is still the best single refusal method, you can use other refusal strategies:

- Suggest an alternative activity that does not involve substance use (e.g., 'Let's go bowling, play hoops, play video games, go to the movies'; 'Let's go to the coffee shop').
- Ask that the person(s) offering change his/her/their behavior (e.g., 'Don't ask me to use').
- Avoid arguing, debating, or giving vague answers.
- Offer legitimate excuses (e.g., 'I can't get into trouble again'; 'I know I am going to have a pee test soon').
- Tell the person(s) about treatment ('Using is a problem for me, so I am in treatment to quit using—I am asking you to help me by not asking me to use again, thanks').
- Leave the situation or stay away from the high-risk situation in the first place—being with using friends."

Skill-Use Guidelines: Modeling and Role Playing

DEMONSTRATION EXERCISE 1

Ask an adolescent to name high-risk use situations that trigger urges and craving; the clinician demonstrates the use of several techniques for dealing with the cravings and urges.

DEMONSTRATION EXERCISE 2

Adolescents offer the clinician drugs or alcohol; the clinician offers refusal responses.

In each of these exercises, the clinician or another adolescent first models a substance-avoiding response; then the adolescent can practice similar responses. For example: A friend is calling the adolescent on the phone, asking if he or she wants to go downtown.

ADOLESCENT (*playing the part of a peer*): Hey, let's go downtown. A lot of folks are hanging around in the park. Lots of weed!

CLINICIAN (*playing the part of a peer*): Nah, I've got to get up early.

ADOLESCENT: As if . . . ! I can come over; I think my brother will give me some weed—and some beer he has.

CLINICIAN: No can do. I have a lot of work tomorrow.

TEEN GROUP EXERCISE 1

Some adolescents take turns presenting a high-risk situation, and other adolescents take turns responding with techniques for dealing with cravings and urges. Examples include (1) The adolescent is offered marijuana or alcohol at a party, (2) a peer asks the adolescent to skip a class, and (3) a peer asks the adolescent over to hang out. Adolescents can come up with realistic situations.

TEEN GROUP EXERCISE 2

Adolescents take turns offering other teens drugs or alcohol, who offer refusal responses.

In a group setting with multiple adolescents, the peers act as a reality check in that they can critique the realistic nature of the situation and the response. The clinician, along with observing adolescents, can coach the teen involved in the exercise. With each exercise, the clinician should "debrief" participating adolescents as to how they felt during the exercise and whether they could make a positive response in real life.

Homework and Real-Life Practice Exercises

- Ask each adolescent to develop a personalized craving plan to use in response to cravings/urges to use.
- Review triggers list.
- Keep a craving/urges log, along with a triggers log, until the next session.

Session 4: Crisis Control: Planning for Lapses and Other Emergencies

Session Outline

- Debrief: Review of past week and relevant interim concerns.
- Review of practice homework.
- Introducing the planning for lapses.

- Planning for emergencies.
  - □ Deal with triggers at once.
  - □ Leave the situation.
  - □ Get rid of the drugs or alcohol.
  - □ Call someone for help.
- Skill-use guidelines—Modeling and role playing.
- Group exercises.
  - □ Exercise 1: Previous lapse experiences.
  - □ Exercise 2: Develop an emergency plan.
- Homework.
  - □ Develop a personalized emergency lapse and relapse plan.
  - □ Keep trigger, cravings, and urges log.

Review of Client Status

Review general functioning and activities, substance use triggers encountered and responses, and use of skills.

Review of Practice Homework

Review personalized craving plans, practice refusal skills, and review modified triggers log with urges and cravings.

Introducing Planning for Lapses

Understanding relapse requires understanding its specific meaning. A single instance of substance use is not defined as a relapse. It is a "lapse," which is a momentary slip or limited instance of substance use. Relapse is a return to a previous *pattern* of use or repeated use. Relapse is thought to be multidetermined, influenced by self-efficacy, outcome expectancies, craving, motivation, coping, emotional states, and interpersonal factors. In view of research on predictors of positive adolescent SUD outcomes following treatment, the clinician should target the following variables during treatment: self-efficacy, negative outcome expectancies, coping skills and their use following treatment, positive affect, and functional social support.

Again, identification and vigilance about recognizing triggers early are critical to decreasing the chances for a lapse or relapse. The triggers for lapse/relapse are almost the same as those for thoughts, urges, and cravings. When lapses occur, they may be accompanied by feelings of guilt and shame. These feelings must be dealt with at once, before they lead to a true relapse. After a slip, one should try to learn, from the events that preceded it, to reduce the likelihood of a repetition. The *abstinence violation effect* occurs when an adolescent, having made a personal commitment to abstain from using a substance, has an initial lapse. Feelings of guilt and hopelessness then act as a further precipitant to triggering an actual relapse.

Planning for Emergencies

It is not a question of whether lapses will happen but of when they will happen and what the adolescent will do in response. Adolescents need to have plans for dealing with thoughts, urges and cravings, high-risk situations, lapses, and relapses. The plan can take the form of the typical CBT techniques described in earlier sessions, but there should also be an emergency plan. Strategies can include using problem-solving skills, calling people for support, increasing attendance at self-help group meetings (e.g., AA, Alateen), and adopting relapse-prevention strategies. The plan should provide as much specific detail as possible (e.g., names, phone numbers, locations of meetings). Some specific guidelines for dealing with the immediate aftermath of a substance use episode include leaving the situation and setting in which the substance use occurred. The adolescent should get rid of the drug(s) or alcohol and call someone for help (AA/NA sponsor, a friend, clinician, or the treatment program).

Lapses may be useful as a teaching moment, underscoring the risks of recovery. It's useful to do a functional analysis of the lapse and relapse. Look at possible triggers, including the "who," "when," and "where" of the situation, and anticipatory thoughts. Were there expectations that substance use would change something or meet some need? Reactions to the episode should also be analyzed, including behavior, thoughts, and feelings, with special attention to feelings of guilt, depression, and self-blame. Catastrophizing thoughts, such as "It's hopeless or "I'll never change," are common reactions that, unchecked, can contribute to further use. Discussing these episodes will help the adolescent to plan more effective coping responses, renew the commitment to abstinence, and view such incidents as learning opportunities.

> "Identify high-risk situations and triggers that might increase the risk of a lapse or relapse."
> "Prepare an emergency plan for coping with stress, other triggers, and the lapse."
> "If you use, stop; remove yourself from the situation and call for help."
> "Complete a functional analysis with your clinician."

Skill-Use Guidelines: Modeling and Role Playing

DEMONSTRATION EXERCISE 1

Adolescents present lapse/relapse situations for the clinician's response.

Group Exercises

EXERCISE 1: PREVIOUS LAPSE EXPERIENCES

Ask about the adolescents' previous experience with lapses or relapses. What worked and what did not?

EXERCISE 2: DEVELOP AN EMERGENCY PLAN

Have the group develop an emergency plan.

Homework and Real-Life Practice Exercises

- Develop a personalized emergency and lapse/relapse plan.
- Keep trigger, cravings, and urges log.

Other Skills Topics

Several other versions of CBT for adolescent SUDs have covered a wider range of topics. Once a clinician has sufficient experience with the core sessions, inclusion of these other topics on a regular or elective basis is feasible. Many of these topics deal with communication and interpersonal and parental conflict. The latter topic is part of the behavioral family intervention described in the next chapter. Clinicians can prepare adolescents for the family intervention by teaching them communication skills, acquainting them with adaptive strategies, encouraging self-efficacy, and enhancing motivation to participate. This adolescent prelude to the family intervention increases the chances that the joint exercises practiced will be successful.

Interpersonal Conflict

Not surprisingly, adolescents, particularly those with problems such as SUDs and other psychiatric disorders, commonly get into conflict with those around them such as parents, siblings, and friends. Poor relationships with parents is a risk factor and is often seen in teens with SUDs. Conflict is also a common consequence of substance use as parents, peers, and others may be upset about the adolescent's use or consequences of use—poor grades, other deviant behavior, and irresponsibility. Conflict affects communication. In the next chapter, we discuss communication as a critical component of family-based interventions. Parents must be willing to talk—and listen—to their adolescent while the adolescent has the same responsibility. Communication skills, especially as they relate to parents and parental conflict, are discussed in more detail in the next chapter.

Criticism

In clinical situations, I find that adolescents have a difficult time dealing with the criticism that their behavior has inevitably invited. However, if given and received appropriately, criticism provides us with a valuable chance to learn things about ourselves and about how we affect other people. Constructive feedback from others helps us to make positive changes in ourselves. Another reason to practice receiving criticism gracefully is that doing so helps teens to avoid unnecessary arguments and lets other people know that they may be receptive to hearing their point of view. In contrast, the person who responds angrily to criticism will discourage others from speaking up again, which may lead to more conflict as well as more serious consequences in the future.

One of the goals of CBT is training the adolescent to discern constructive criticism and make receptive and assertive responses. Interpersonal conflicts resulting in anger or other negative feelings are high-risk situations for relapse. Failure to respond effectively to criticism can lead to serious interpersonal conflicts, whereas having an effective response can reduce conflicts and the probability of substance use.

Sometimes criticism about drinking or substance use will take the form of accusations or inquiries—for example, "You're home late. I know you've been drinking again." It is important to be able to respond to statements like this in a way that facilitates productive communication and does not start a fight. Even if the criticism is delivered in a nonconstructive manner, the adolescent can learn to respond assertively and effectively. Sometimes the criticism about substance use will focus on past events or on the negative consequences of past drinking. However the criticism is phrased, it is important to respond effectively and to focus on here-and-now solutions without getting sidetracked into a nonproductive rehashing of past conflicts.

When the adolescent receives criticism, he or she should be prompted to do or not do the following:

- Don't respond in a negative manner; don't debate or counterattack.
- Find something to agree with in the criticism.

- Ask questions for clarification.
- Propose a workable compromise.

Increasing Prosocial Behaviors and Peer Relationships

Although most CM studies have concentrated on increasing abstinence from specific illicit drugs, some CM studies in adults have focused on increasing other behaviors consistent with addiction recovery recommendations. One particular class of behavior involves reinforcing prosocial activities and compliance with treatment goals consistent with a drug-free lifestyle. CM can also be arranged to reinforce attendance at outpatient counseling or recovery groups and to encourage prosocial activities as a constructive way to replace the time spent using alcohol and other drugs. Specifically for adolescents, increasing prosocial and personal goal-related activities has several potential advantages, including the following:

- Scheduling activities at times when adolescents might otherwise use alcohol or other drugs.
- Participating in activities that expose adolescents to nonusing peers, thus decreasing the likelihood of use.
- Developing healthier peer group affiliations.
- Developing new leisure interests or rekindling old ones that increase life satisfaction without alcohol or drugs.
- Increasing activities with parents and other family members.
- Increasing participation in treatment, 12-step meetings, and other recovery-oriented programs.

The idea of reinforcing client-initiated activities is consistent with several evidence-based approaches evaluated with adolescents and could serve as a useful adjunct to improve adherence to therapies, such as A-CRA, described in Chapter 5, and MET/CBT (Sampl & Kadden, 2001).

Unfortunately, identifying prosocial activities and peers is easier said than done. Adolescents with SUDs often have deficits that result in poor peer relations (e.g., impulsivity, poor social problem solving), especially with prosocial peers. In order to increase prosocial behavior, I suggest a behavioral approach by reinforcing positive behavior. This type of reinforcement involves several steps.

1. *Identify the long-term positive consequences of the prosocial behavior.* Spend time with the adolescent probing this topic to identify what the adolescent finds reinforcing. Behaviors or activities that are reinforcing in many different areas of the adolescent's life, such as those listed next, can compete with using drugs (Meyers & Smith, 1995). The clinician might

ask, "What are the positive results of [specific prosocial activity] in each of these areas?"

- Family members.
- Friends.
- Physical feelings.
- Emotional feelings.
- Legal situations.
- School situations.
- Job situations.
- Financial situations.
- Other situations.

This technique is similar to the decisional balance technique in MI, but it's more focused on the positive consequences of prosocial behaviors. When adolescents consider the positive aspects of their behavior on their lives and other people in their lives, they also reflect on the negative consequences of their past and future behaviors.

   2. *Use a happiness scale.* Another similar method of reinforcing the positive consequences of prosocial behavior is the use of a "happiness scale" to assess how happy or satisfied an adolescent is in multiple life areas. These life areas include his or her use or nonuse of alcohol or drugs, relationships with friends and boyfriends or girlfriends, relationships with parents or caregivers, school, social activities, recreational activities, personal habits, legal issues, money management, emotional well-being, communication, and general happiness. A *happiness scale* or survey completed early in treatment shows the areas of an adolescent's life that are most in need of attention. Although the happiness scale can be used as a barometer of progress at any time, one of its important uses is to gather information to help develop a comprehensive treatment plan.

   In CBT, clinicians can help adolescents learn how to increase their prosocial recreational activities to involve nonusing acquaintances by:

- Recognizing that being in a situation where they used in the past puts them at risk for relapse.
- Identifying prosocial activities to try.
- Understanding how to make initial contacts for the new activities.
- Identifying and enlisting support persons who can meet or accompany the adolescent to the new activity.
- Becoming committed to sampling new, prosocial activities.
- Selecting a new activity to try as part of the homework assignment.

Adolescents in SUD treatment usually have developed many social and recreational activities centered on the use of alcohol or drugs. It is therefore normal for youth to find it difficult to find new drug-free activities or friends. Because both adults and youth with drug problems have devoted much of their free time to getting high, they need to reengage in positive leisure activities to find a drug-free life rewarding. Emphasize to the adolescent that everyone wants to have fun but that there are ways to have fun other than getting high. Encourage the adolescent to believe that together the therapist and the adolescent can find other ways to have fun.

3. *Know recreational resources in the community.* Become familiar with a wide variety of recreational resources available in your community and develop lists of potential activities (see Figure 6.5). These lists can be developed by adolescents in youth groups, in health classes in high schools, in groups of adolescents participating in substance abuse treatment, or in other groups of adolescents who are easily accessible. Review Figure 6.3 to have a better understanding of the triggers and consequences of prosocial behavior that an adolescent may already be participating in. To do these procedures well, continually update your knowledge about community resources that provide fun and positive recreational activities (reinforcers). Good sources of information about these activities are local newspapers, youth groups, and service agencies.

4. *Reinforcer sampling.* A primary method to help adolescents increase prosocial activities is to help them try out or sample new activities. When adolescents do so, they experience a time-out from using drugs and begin to appreciate the positive benefits of such prosocial activities and abstinence. Deviant behaviors, including substance use and behaviors associated with use, are disrupted, and there is an opportunity to replace them with new, positive coping skills.

In discussions of new prosocial activities with the adolescent, be both positive and encouraging. Explain that you understand that he or she will, at times, miss previous activities but that reverting to old habits may bring back serious problems or may start the teen on a path toward serious problems. Searching for new, positive recreational outlets that are incompatible with drug use is a key component of the adolescent community reinforcement approach (A-CRA; Godley et al., 2001). In fact, the underlying theory of the A-CRA is that it helps adolescents create a drug-free lifestyle that is so rewarding that they would not want to return to drug use and perhaps lose all that they have achieved (e.g., improved family relationships, newfound friends, discovered fun activities).

Sampling new activities provides an opportunity to build rapport. It enables adolescents to set goals that are reasonable and attainable. Meeting these goals promotes their self-efficacy—the belief that they can complete certain tasks. When people believe they can follow through with one task, they are usually more successful in following through with other tasks. Self-efficacy can be generalized to the task of staying substance free. The clinician should become acquainted with the prosocial activities available in the adolescent's community and school.

Getting an adolescent to try out a new social or recreational outlet may be challenging. One way to encourage this activity is to frame it as sampling. That is, encourage the adolescent to try it once to see whether there is any potential for enjoying it. For example, you might say, "You mentioned you liked cars. Would you like to go to a car show to see what one is like?"

5. *Use prosocial activities to compete with high-risk occasions.* The functional analysis of substance use provides knowledge about an adolescent's pattern of drug use (e.g., weekend use). These times are the high-risk occasions for using; make these times the primary targets for new recreational alternatives, although even within participation in prosocial activities, the adolescent may be exposed to various high-risk situations. Review high-risk situations (people, places, and things) to set the stage for helping the adolescent to replace these occasions with positive activities.

"You mentioned you don't want to smoke weed during the next month, and weekends are a high-risk time. Is there some activity that you can think of that will be fun to do during the weekends that does not involve alcohol or drugs? This way you don't have to worry about being put in detention or about your mom getting upset."

Keep in mind that many adolescents have little ability to socially interact with non-drug-using peers. Most of their prior social interactions may have been centered on the drug culture, and drug use may have been a social lubricant for them. So you may need to refer to communication training procedures to help them learn how to make conversation in new groups.

Encourage the adolescent to engage in several new activities that build on each new success. The adolescent is likely to get more out of social occasions if he or she engages in them frequently and makes an effort to be part of the group activities and conversation. For example, if the teen joins a youth group, he or she is more likely to feel a sense of belonging to the group and make friends more easily by attending activities weekly rather than monthly.

6. *Enlist social support.* You might ask, "Who are the people who don't want you to smoke weed? Who will help you stay straight?" Whenever

Recreational Activities	Leisure Activities	Hobbies
Backpacking	Attending auctions	Amateur radio
Baseball/softball	Attending auto races	Aquarium making
Basketball	Attending concerts	Arts and crafts
Billiards/playing pool	Attending plays	Astronomy
Bowling	Attending sports events	Auto repairing
Camping	Bicycling	Carpentry
Canoeing	Bird watching	Ceramics/pottery
Checkers	Coin collecting	Coaching Little League
Chess	Crossword puzzles	Computers
Dancing	Dining out	Cooking/baking
Golf/mini-golf	Driving	Electronics
Ice skating	Fishing	Flower arranging
Playing cards	Hiking	Gardening
Sailing/boating	Horseback riding	Genealogy
Shuffleboard	Listening to music	Home decorating
Skiing	Painting	Hunting
Skindiving	Picnics	Model building
Surfboarding	Playing video games	Photography
Swimming	Reading books	Playing music
Table tennis	Roller skating	Sewing
Touch football	Sightseeing	Singing
Volleyball	Sunbathing	Stained glass making
Weightlifting	Talking to friends	Volunteering
Make/fly paper airplanes	Visiting museums	Woodworking
Collect bugs	Walks in parks	Writing a story
Wash car(s)	Watching movies and TV	Writing a song
Write in journal	Writing	Creating a website

FIGURE 6.5. What can I do? Adapted from Center for Substance Abuse Treatment (1999b).

possible, identify a support person who can meet or accompany the adolescent to the new activity. This should lessen nervousness about participation and help increase commitment to attending because the adolescent knows someone is expecting him or her.

If an adolescent says he or she is willing to try a new activity, explore possible obstacles to trying it and present problem-solving techniques, if needed, to determine whether the activity presents any risk from potential triggers. Ask the adolescent to identify a good time to try the activity, and get him or her to make a commitment to actually carry it out. Advise the adolescent that it may be easier to participate in structured activities (e.g., a skating party) than go to a party. Stress that participation in new activities becomes easier with practice.

An activity list that provides telephone numbers is particularly helpful when sampling new behaviors. To encourage the adolescent to find out more about an activity, you may ask him or her to make a telephone call using the list during the session. Before doing so, you should work with the adolescent to develop a list of questions that are appropriate and then role-play a typical information-seeking call. It is also appropriate to assign additional calls for homework. Provide encouragement throughout, and praise any successes.

7. *Systematic encouragement.* Because it may be difficult for adolescents to engage in a variety of new prosocial activities, Meyers and Smith (1995) recommend three steps for encouraging adolescents: brainstorming, role playing, and providing feedback.

Never assume that an adolescent will make a first contact independently. Brainstorm, role-play, and give feedback to the adolescent upon making the initial contact. Brainstorming would center on obtaining information about how to access an activity. You might say, "You said you would like to try rock climbing; how can we find a place to learn how to do this?" You may need to use a problem-solving procedure to help the adolescent figure out how to access an activity.

When role playing, it is important to encourage the adolescent's participation. Although role playing can be somewhat awkward for some people, it is an important part of encouraging the adolescent to try new activities because it helps him or her visualize and actually carry out what you are asking. When possible, observe the adolescent making the initial phone call. You can observe how well the adolescent performs this activity and provide reinforcement for taking this positive step.

8. *Review the experience.* Review the experience in the next session to determine its reinforcement value. (The activity can serve as a form of homework.)

General Skills Associated with Substance Use Problems

Many CBT programs for SUDs include several skills that do not deal specifically with substance use. Instead they target deficits that frequently occur with substance use problems. Many of these skills are collected under a general rubric of problem-solving or coping skills and include anger awareness and control, awareness and management of negative thinking, negative moods, and depression. The latter skills tie SUD CBT with its older sibling CBT for depression or anxiety. Clinicians can use other CBT modules to target problems such as suicidal ideation and behavior, anxiety, emotion regulation, interpersonal effectiveness, and distress tolerance skills. I will not review these areas, but I want to emphasize the need to tie these issues, when relevant to the individual adolescent's presenting problems, to the adolescent's substance use as much as possible. For additional information on such modules, the reader is referred to other sources: Brent, Poling, and Goldstein, 2011; Kennard, Hughes, and Foxwell, 2016; Rathus and Miller, 2014.

Troubleshooting

Treatment Resistance

Treatment resistance is most often regarded as a problem with the adolescent's or the parents' motivation and denial. However, treatment resistance can also mean lack of success in obtaining abstinence, decreasing substance use, or improving function. Of those adolescents entering SUD treatment, 20–25% either never change their level of use or deteriorate over time after achieving some decreased use. The good news is that more than half achieve abstinence rapidly or slowly improve, decreasing use over time. I have already discussed the issue of what to do with unmotivated adolescents. As long as they come to treatment, intervention strategies should continue such as maintaining communication, using motivational techniques, using parents as agents of change, and allowing natural consequences.

The most salient aspect of motivation is respect for the adolescent's autonomy; the clinician cannot make the adolescent participate in treatment. The clinician can avoid resistance and potentially increase engagement by assuming a collaborative, nonjudgmental attitude. Avoid confrontation and attempt to understand any ambivalence that the adolescent has about engaging in some type of treatment with some type of goal for treatment. Although an MI approach may resolve enough of the adolescent's ambivalence and lead to some degree of participation in treatment, sometimes it does not. In such cases, the clinician may facilitate the use of some contingencies described in Chapter 2, such as the loss of privileges at home, placement consequences if the adolescent is involved in the juvenile justice system, or treatment commitment, depending on state law. These methods apply whether the adolescent is considering entry into treatment or exhibits highly resistant behavior during the course of treatment. If such leverage to participate does not exist or work, the clinician should work with the parents to improve their communication skills, monitoring and supervision, and contingency management (see Chapter 7). Periodically during a parent-oriented treatment, the clinician should regularly invite the adolescent into treatment to represent his or her own interests in designing a system of rules, consequences, reinforcers, and contracts.

The clinician should assist parents in not rescuing their teen and should allow the adolescent to receive any natural consequences of his or her behavior (e.g., arrests and juvenile justice placements, school sanctions).

"Tom, I know that you feel that you don't have a problem. But both you and your parents have reported a lot of conflict—arguing and fighting at home. I would at least like to help you improve what's going on at home. You have indicated that you do not want to be a part of treatment, and I cannot make you. But your parents want to make things better for you and them at home, so I am going to work with them to help them communicate better with you and make reasonable rules, consequences, and rewards. Of course, I would like to see your interests represented. I will do my best, but it would be better if you could participate even a bit. So let me know if you change your mind or if there is something else we can do to help you."

What about the adolescent who just does not improve or does not improve enough? The reasons can range from poor motivation, poor compliance, and impulsivity to poor problem solving. Regardless of the reason, several steps are suggested.

1. Reassess family functioning.
2. Change level of care.
3. Check motivational approach.
4. Check status of comorbid psychiatric disorder(s).
5. Check recovery skills.
6. Check prosocial environment.

The Highly Resistant Teen

There are several populations of youth who are more likely to be treatment resistant. These include more deviant youth, especially those involved with illegal activities such as gangs and drug dealing; those with long-standing problems with aggression, dysregulated behavior, and emotions; and those with opiate or substance dependence, especially methamphetamine and IV drug use. For the last group, the addictive powers of the substances often seem intractable. Treatment professionals often find they need comprehensive approaches over a long period of acute treatment and aftercare. The availability of replacement medications such as buprenorphine for opiate withdrawal, short-term acute treatment, and maintenance treatment should prompt the inclusion of such medications in a comprehensive treatment plan after no more than one or two attempts at drug-free therapy.

The Frequent Relapser

Relapse is common among adolescents with moderate to severe SUDs. Many clinicians and parents become frustrated when abstinence is not maintained, which they consider treatment failure. But this is not necessarily the case. Clinicians need to consider the following:

■ Is this a true relapse—a return to a previous pattern of use—or a lapse that might quickly be corrected back to abstinence or minimal use? Assuming a lapse is a full relapse can invite the abstinence violation effect and make relapse more likely. The adolescent, parents, and clinician should not rush to judgment or become unduly upset before the context of the substance use episode is considered. How long has the adolescent been abstinent or otherwise improving in treatment? What are the goals and reasonable expectations of treatment—for example, harm reduction with reduced psychosocial impairment and improved functioning?

■ If this is a true relapse, what contingencies are in place for the adolescent? The consequences for the adolescent's substance use should have been considered and set early in treatment.

■ What is necessary to get the adolescent back on track? A booster skills session? A different modality? For example, if the previous treatment was CBT, then family therapy or a higher level of care such as acute residential or long-term residential treatment might be tried next. Should there be improvement in community support such as access to prosocial activities and peer groups and reevaluation of the school situation?

■ If this is opiate use disorder, does the adolescent need maintenance medication such as buprenorphine?

■ Is psychiatric comorbidity a factor? Consider reevaluation of emotional and behavioral symptoms and referral, or evaluation for appropriate psychotherapies and/or medication.

Applying a chronic disease model to SUDs suggests that relapses can be expected. Clinicians and treatment programs should develop and maintain the capacity to manage relapse and chronicity through such methods as changing and/or broadening the intervention mix for an individual adolescent and, above all, not dismissing the adolescent due to relapse. As long as adolescents and their families come to treatment, they should be welcomed and treated.

SUMMARY

To change their substance use behaviors, adolescents generally require additional skills. CBT for adolescents with SUDs provides these skills through a functional analysis of substance use behaviors and skill building. These strategies emphasize identifying and anticipating "triggers," that is, the people, places, and things that prompt use, thoughts about use, and cravings. Skills building includes management of thoughts and cravings about substance use, problem solving, and creating plans to deal with lapses and relapse. Additional skills might include dealing with interpersonal conflict, stress, depression, anxiety and other negative emotions. CBT for SUD emphasizes the development and maintenance of a positive support network of prosocial peers, parents, and other adults. As peer factors account for some of the risk for developing and maintaining substance use and SUDs, peer-based interventions can be important elements of overall treatment for adolescents with SUDs. Peer-based interventions include group-based CBT, 12-step work, AA/NA meetings, and just having fun with nonusing peers. Many peer-based interventions can be seen as adjuncts to family- and skills-based interventions and as an important element of aftercare where ultimate success may hinge on development of a prosocial peer group and participation in prosocial activities.

Chapter Seven

Parent Management Training

Family interventions are critical to the success of most treatment approaches for adolescents with SUDs. A number of family-related risk factors have been identified for the development of substance use and SUDs among adolescents. Four domains of predictors have figured prominently in longitudinal studies of the etiology of adolescent substance use and SUDs: poor parent–adolescent relationship; ineffective parental discipline; adolescent abuse and neglect; and parental alcoholism or other parental SUDs.

Although there are many specific approaches to family intervention for substance abuse treatment, they have several common goals: (1) providing psychoeducation about SUDs, which decreases familial resistance to treatment and increases motivation and engagement; (2) assisting parents and family to initiate and maintain efforts to get the adolescent into appropriate treatment and achieve abstinence; (3) assisting parents and family to establish or reestablish structure with consistent limit setting, careful monitoring, and supervision of the adolescent's activities and behavior; (4) improving communication among family members; and (5) getting other family members into treatment and/or support programs as needed.

Family therapy is the most studied modality in the treatment of adolescents with SUDs. As discussed in Chapter 1, forms of family therapy that have the support of controlled studies are functional family therapy, brief strategic family therapy, multisystemic therapy, family systems therapy, and multidimensional family therapy. An integrated behavioral and family therapy model that combines a family systems model and CBT also appears to be efficacious. The research supporting family modalities is also found in Chapter 1.

Learning and administering specific family therapies requires both grounding in general therapeutic approaches and specific training in the particular family therapy model. The family therapy model almost always includes ongoing supervision. This often highly specific training is not always available to clinicians. While a detailed description of each model and its specific training is beyond the scope of this chapter, I review some basic principles of family therapy and specific issues relevant to adolescents with SUDs and their families and offer a model of behavioral family therapy.

ELEMENTS OF A FAMILY-BASED BEHAVIORAL THERAPY

A review of family models used for the treatment of adolescents with SUDs suggests several critical elements for successful family interventions: (1) parent and adolescent motivation and engagement, (2) parent management training (PMT), (3) communication skills, and (4) problem-solving skills for the family as a whole.

Using these elements, Brooke Molina of the University of Pittsburgh and I developed a family-based model, initially for younger adolescents with high-risk behaviors but applicable to older adolescents and their families with substance use-related behaviors. Parent training, usually in a group of parents, leads to improvements in various target behaviors. But parent training alone is often less effective with adolescents than with younger children. Therefore, our family-based behavioral therapy has three main parts:

1. PMT, covered in this chapter.
2. Communication training for parents, which may be delivered as part of PMT, and communication skills for adolescents, which may be part of recovery skills training (Chapter 6).
3. Parent–adolescent problem solving in joint sessions (covered in Chapter 8).

Each of these parts may be delivered together as part of a more comprehensive intervention approach, alone, or in combinations that befit the needs of the adolescent and his or her family.

This chapter focuses on PMT. The problem-solving and communications skills learned by parents in PMT are used during parent–adolescent problem solving, which includes negotiation skills training. To maximize the effectiveness of the parenting sessions, we place an emphasis on reasonable or achievable goals for parenting behavior change. For example, negotiating curfew times and monitoring the whereabouts of adolescents are more attainable goals than prohibition of any outside activities and making straight A's on the next report card in school. The order of specific session topics should be flexible to allow maximum attention to parental goals and concerns.

Parent Self-Efficacy and Motivation

PMT teaches parents new skills. To learn new skills, parents have to have both motivation and the capacity to learn. Often, parents' previous efforts and limited skills are futile in controlling their adolescent, and so the primary goal for family-based services is to change a pattern of ineffective and/or coercive parenting practices. However, parents are generally very sensitive when their parenting is explicitly and implicitly questioned during the course of treatment; they become defensive about current discipline strategies when confronted directly. Motivation to change parental behaviors is hindered by self-protective attributions ("Our son's behavior is the problem, not us"), lack of experience with praise and nonpunitive discipline strategies, and limited faith that alternative methods will result in improved adolescent behavior. Openness in discussing the pros and cons of a variety of parenting strategies, developing an understanding of core parenting values and beliefs, and avoiding confrontations on corporal punishment may help reduce defensiveness (Chaffin et al., 2004).

Motivation cannot be assumed. Despite the often extreme difficulties presented by their adolescent, parents may not be motivated to participate in PMT or communication skills. Parents may have had a negative treatment experience, or they may have a negative attitude about treatment itself or a particular type of treatment. Although PMT is often seen as a directive, structured form of therapy, the clinician will often have to be flexible in conducting sessions to gain and maintain parental engagement and motivation. Skills training for families requires commitment, willingness to work, consistency, tenacity, tolerance for the frustration of learning any new idea or skill, and a sense of self-efficacy, which makes the attempt seem other than futile and defeating.

Parents may be less likely to react with frustration and abusive acts if they have an accurate understanding of adolescent development and appropriate expectations for behavior. However, preconceived ideas about development are often closely held and based on advice from other family members or other parenting role models. Parents may hold inappropriate assumptions about the adolescent's ability to control impulses, sustain self-control, or remember and perform multiple or complex directives. The clinician's direct education and correction may be met with defensiveness, reducing the positive impact of the information. MI strategies may be helpful in generating openness to new information by encouraging parents to identify areas where gaps in their knowledge may exist.

PARENT 1: We try to ground him, but he usually has no privileges, nothing to take away. He often ignores punishment and comes home late—not even stopping by after school. My family thinks we are too easy on him, that we should send him away or have him arrested, turn him in to the police. I know he probably has pot in his room.

CLINICIAN: It is very difficult knowing what to do. It sounds like you have really tried your best to help Bobby and you feel kind of helpless—and maybe hopeless, too. You mentioned that you have children who are successful in school and do not appear to get into trouble—so you are a good parent. But Bobby is a challenging kid. He is impulsive and appears to be a poor problem solver. You need some extra skills that are tailored to help set some limits on some of Bobby's bad behavior.

PARENT 2: We have tried. At this point, he just ignores us and does what he wants.

CLINICIAN: I know you have made a big effort. In solving some of these problems and setting limits, Bobby has to be able to believe he has some say in what he can do. He has to be able to make some mistakes without digging himself too deep in a hole with punishments. And there have to be rewards for positive behaviors—no matter how little they seem. At this point, he has to think you are at least sometimes listening to him and his viewpoint. And even if you send him away, before long you will be back trying to decide how to make rules and set limits that will be effective in controlling his unwanted behaviors. If it is OK with you, we can review some goals that other parents have found reasonable.

When you do make rules, the rules should be realistic. Rather than getting straight A's, maybe attending school, homework completion, and improvement in grades are more reasonable short-term goals. Can you think of some rules like that?

PARENT 1: Maybe we can start with those goals. But I also want to know where Bobby is, where he is going.

PARENT 2: He needs to be respectful when he talks with us. Of course, we do not want him using drugs.

For the most part, the clinician uses MI techniques such as OARS. In the above example, the clinician first expresses empathy with the parent: "It is very difficult knowing what to do." The clinician then sees evidence to explicitly say, "You are a good parent" to help build parent self-efficacy. Only then does the clinician begin to offer "extra skills" given the "challenging kid." Finally, the clinician asks for permission to provide information about reasonable goals and provides a menu of possible goals from which the parents can select what is appropriate for them.

PMT FOR PARENTS OF ADOLESCENTS WITH SUDs

PMT for parents of adolescents with SUDs is based on a social learning and operant behavioral model. In this first phase of the behavioral family therapy model, a group of parents and other caregivers meet without their adolescents. Sessions focus on (1) identifying parent concerns and goals for treatment; (2) psychoeducation about PMT principles, techniques, and strategies; (3) development of a functional analysis of deviant adolescent behaviors as they relate to current parent management practices; (4) parents learning specific PMT strategies as they relate to parent-identified goals; (5) improvement of parent–adolescent communication; and (6) preparation for parent–adolescent therapy sessions, which involve family problem solving and improving communication.

Optimally, PMT is delivered in a group setting of parents (optimally, three to eight sets of parents) so that they can share experiences and learn that others have similar problems. PMT can be delivered to individual families as well. When two-parent households are involved, the presence of both parents is often critical to minimizing inconsistency in parenting. Others such as grandparents or other family members who act in the parental role should also be involved. Sessions in the group format generally last 90 minutes, and those in the individual format last 45 minutes. The number of sessions is somewhat variable, depending on the baseline skills of the parent(s) and the behavioral goal(s). Weekly sessions balance parents' need for quick improvement with time for parents to practice their new skills at home. Rarely are more than eight sessions necessary to deliver PMT's basic elements. In addition, booster or follow-up sessions may be scheduled to review progress and past lessons or to make midcourse corrections. Midweek phone call appointments can be used to check on progress at home and problem solve failed attempts at behavior change, school-related difficulties, and effective communication with school staff. For those in group settings, a few individual family sessions are useful to deal with issues and problems specific to that family.

Session Structure

The general structure of the sessions is consistent across sessions, as shown in Table 7.1. Similar to adolescent skills training (Chapter 5), sessions begin with a review of events, specific concerns, behavior, progress (or its lack) since the last session, and any homework that was assigned. A short discussion of a specific topic follows. The clinician should use modeling and role playing to allow parent(s) to practice and to check their understanding of the behavioral task or principle. Finally, homework, in the form of a specific task or practice, is assigned to be reviewed at the next session.

Although a clinician can deliver PMT for adolescents and their families as a stand-alone intervention, I recommend concurrent involvement in parent–adolescent negotiation and adolescent skills training. Many of the parent management skills and resulting household rules discussed in this chapter do require some degree of adolescent compliance or "buy-in."

Session Topics

In PMT sessions, the following topics can be covered as needed:

1. Explanation of PMT, goal setting, adolescent development, and the development of substance use disorders.
2. Parental monitoring and tracking of the adolescent's behavior as a means to (a) decrease substance use and rule-breaking behavior, (b) understand the antecedents and consequences of problem behaviors, including substance use and abuse, and (c) assist with management of the environment to decrease exposure to drug stimuli and drug craving.
3. Discipline, rules, and negative consequences.
4. Contingency management, including the development of positive and negative consequences.
5. Effective communication with teenagers and problem-solving techniques.
6. Introduce contracts to parent–adolescent problem solving.

TABLE 7.1. General Session Format for Behavioral Family Therapy

1. Review of week's activities, progress, and problems.
2. Review and discussion of homework.
3. Presentation of new content area and discussion of relevance to the adolescent.
4. Modeling and role-play practice.
5. Assignment of homework.

The Role of the Professional

Ideally, parents learn how to manage their adolescents through skills attainment, which involves setting goals, negotiating rules, and practice—both in session and at home. The clinician's role involves engaging the adolescent and his or her parents through an understanding and demonstration of the process, as well as practice of the process. In a group setting, parents assist each other in a role similar to that of the clinician, but the clinician provides additional "expert" commentary about the process and maintains the overall structure of each session.

Session 1: Introductions, Explanation of PMT, Goal Setting and Adolescent Development

Session Outline

- Introductions: clinician, parents.
- Determining goals for therapy: What do the parents want to change?
  - □ What are the parents' specific goals and expectations?
  - □ Providing an overview and rationale for this treatment.
    - Establishing the parental role.
    - Developing rules, rewards for compliance and good behavior, and consequences for undesirable behavior.
  - □ Assessing parent experience, knowledge, and attitudes about PMT.
  - □ Discussing session procedures, structure, and content (including adolescent sessions and parent–adolescent problem solving).
- Introducing principles for parenting.
  - □ What parents can control and what they cannot.
  - □ Development of substance use behaviors and problems.
    - Genetic risk.
    - Family and other environmental risk factors.
    - Adolescence as a vulnerable period of development.
- What should parents expect of adolescents?
- Homework: Develop a problem list (goals for therapy). Parents should track the occurrence of these problems until the next session.

Introductions

This initial session begins with clinician and parent introductions. Using an MI style, the clinician asks the parents to state their goals and expectations for the treatment. Review of parental goals and aspirations generally center around changes in adolescent behavior in the domains of family, school, and peer functioning.

The clinician then provides an overview of PMT and explains the role of the professional. The clinician should explain the philosophy, goals, and process of the treatment. PMT goals—what the parents are going to learn—are the means by which the parents will attain their goals involving the changes in their adolescent's behavior.

The goals include the establishment of the parental role as outlined in Table 7.2 and the development of positive and negative contingencies for managing the adolescent's behavior. The clinician then reviews the parents' experience with past treatments. He or she should elicit parents' attitudes about the treatment and the parents' confidence in their ability (self-efficacy) to succeed in addressing the treatment goals. If parents have had some experience with parent management techniques, the clinician should attempt to assess their current abilities and confidence level in administering these as well as newer techniques.

Parenting Principles, Overview of Adolescent Development, and SUDs

The clinician then provides psychoeducation about principles of parenting, adolescent development, and the development of SUDs.

"We want our teenagers to be successful adults; therefore, parents should encourage autonomy whenever possible. However, we also need to recognize that adolescents are not ready for full autonomy. The parts of their brains responsible for decision making and planned behavior have not achieved full maturity. That and their hormonal drives prompt risk-taking behavior and undue influence by peers to participate in activities such as substance use. Parents need to provide rules, supervision, and monitoring to prevent the bad behaviors and to promote the good behaviors while understanding that our teens are headed for autonomy, whether or not we like all the aspects of this autonomy."

TABLE 7.2. Establishment of Parental Roles

1. Setting boundary between parent and adolescent.
2. Allowing appropriate independence for the adolescent.
3. Establishing an authoritative supervision style.
4. Establishing rules and consequences.
5. Learning negotiation and communication skills.
6. Focusing on strengths: adolescent and parent abilities.

Development of Substance Use Behaviors

Clinicians should provide some background about how SUDs develop in adolescents. The development of SUDs is a result of a balance of risk and protective factors (see Chapter 1) reflecting a combination of nature and nurture. While we cannot control the increased risk for SUDs in families with SUDs (i.e., the genetic predisposition), we can change some of the environmental risk factors such as parent–adolescent communication, parent monitoring of adolescent activities, reinforcement of prosocial adolescent activities, and adolescent problem solving.

What Should Parents Expect
of Adolescents?

Given the developmental context of SUDs, the clinician should ask what parents should expect from their adolescence—for example, compliance with parental requests (how much?), household rules? home chores? some misbehavior? school and homework?, and, finally, substance use and how much?

Homework

Ask parents to develop a problem list. This list becomes their goals for therapy. Parents should also monitor the occurrence of these problems until the next session by keeping track of the frequency and context of the problem. For example, when during the day or week does each problem behavior occur? Are there precipitants or triggers for these behaviors? How do parents react when these problems occur?

Session 2: Monitoring and Tracking

Session Outline

- Debrief: Review of the past week and relevant interim concerns; review homework.
- Introducing monitoring and tracking adolescent behaviors.
  - Rationale: The importance of monitoring and tracking as a risk factor.
    - Provide structure and expectations of the adolescent.
    - Limit exposure to deviant peers and problem situations.
- Assess parent knowledge, experience in monitoring, and tracking.
- What to monitor: where, who, what, when.

- Provide examples of parent–adolescent interactions, including affect, language, and content.
  - Positive interactions.
  - Negative interactions.
  - Neutral interactions.
- Role plays.
- Homework.
  - Parent–adolescent home conference to review monitoring and tracking rules (may be done in clinician's office).
  - Parent to keep a monitoring/tracking log.

Review the Past Week and Homework

Clinicians should reinforce parents who attempt to complete homework with praise and encourage other parents who do not do the homework. The lesson for last week's homework is for the parent to be mindful of "problems" and to be able to describe the context of these problems as well as have an idea of the frequency of these problems. The clinician should answer any questions and address any problems that parents may have had in doing the homework.

Monitoring and Tracking Behaviors

RATIONALE

Explain that lack of monitoring and supervision is a risk factor for substance use. Parents who monitor their adolescents provide structure and a safe environment.

Ask if parents have any previous experience monitoring or tracking their teen's behaviors.

WHAT TO MONITOR: KEEPING TRACK OF KIDS
(ESPECIALLY WHEN PARENTS NOT AT HOME)

Specific substance use behaviors aside, parents need to always know the following about their teens: *Where* are they? *Who* are they with? *What* are they doing? and *When* will they be home? Parents should know the names of their adolescent's friends, what grade they are in, and how old they are. They should also know their adolescent's friends' addresses, their parent(s)' name(s), as well as if there are any siblings. Ideally, parents should be aware of the kind of persons their friends are, their usual activities and interests, and their reputation.

ADOLESCENT: You never let me hang out with my friends. I should be able to decide what I do with whoever I want.

PARENT: We know you have friends, and we don't want to keep you from having friends and going out with them. But we do have some rules—we need to know where and with whom you are hanging out. We also have limits on how late you are out. Now if there is a good reason for you to be out later, we are willing to listen and consider. If you show you can handle and follow these rules, maybe we can discuss changes later.

In their desire for autonomy, adolescents may legitimately balk about even this level of information about their whereabouts. However, given the ubiquitous cell phone and GPS, this information should be easy to obtain. Although this information is non-negotiable—that is, the teen is expected to comply and provide it with each outside activity—the clinician should encourage parents to reward compliance. What is negotiable is the acceptability of the answers to the parents. In other words, parents must decide for themselves with whom they want their teen to be, where they want them to be going, what they will be doing, and when they are coming home. As the adolescent's overall compliance and behavior improves, the flexibility of the parents should also change.

TRACKING: PAYING ATTENTION TO DETAILS OF THE ADOLESCENT'S BEHAVIOR

To monitor, one must track, that is, account for all behaviors and peers of interest over time, watching for patterns of behavior suggestive of substance use. Where does the teen go? When does he or she go without permission or in defiance of parent rules? How many times is he or she late or on time? In order to ascertain whether the adolescent is improving, that is, whether the undesired behaviors are decreasing and the desired behaviors are increasing, parents need to be able to pay attention and document the behaviors, including the date, time, and situation.

WHAT A PARENT NEEDS TO BE ABLE TO ASK IN ORDER TO BE AN ACTIVE, EFFECTIVE MONITOR

1. *Question:* Who Is My Adolescent With?

    Answer: Know whom your adolescent is hanging out with (i.e., their name).

2. *Question:* What do I know about the person(s) my adolescent is with?

Answer: Know details about the adolescent's friends such as age, where they live, go to school, grade, level of deviant behavior.

3. *Question:* Where is my adolescent?

Answer: Know physically where your adolescent is.

- Develop a system where the adolescent will check in with you so that you know where he or she is or use an electronic means to track.
- The adolescent should report any change in plans or location.

4. *Question:* What is my adolescent doing?

Answer: Know what activity the adolescent is doing, including specific activities or even "hanging out."

5. *Question:* When will my adolescent be leaving and arrive home?

Answer: Know the adolescent's specific schedule of activities and events.

- Establish and enforce a curfew.

Parents should stay informed about their activities and a time-frame of how long those activities should last. Parents should develop a schedule or at least know a head of time who is transporting your adolescent to and/or from the events. Change in plans should prompt a cell phone call (or text) from the adolescent.

Commonly, the adolescent is resistant to such monitoring activities and communication, and so monitoring can be discussed with the adolescent as part of the parent–adolescent negotiation.

Role Plays

Clinician and parents should take turns being "the parent" and "the adolescent." Common scenarios include general monitoring requests about adolescent activity/plans after school and on evenings (weekday and weekend); going to a specific peer's home or a public place; keeping parents informed about changes in plans (e.g., use of cell phones); and curfew.

Homework

- Parent–adolescent home conference to review monitoring and tracking rules (may be done in the clinician's office as part of parent–adolescent negotiation).
- Parent to keep a monitoring/tracking log.

Session 3: Discipline and Negative Consequences

Session 3 Outline

- Debrief: Review of the past week and relevant interim concerns; review of homework.
- Introducing discipline and negative consequences.
  - □ Rationale: The importance of consistent discipline.
  - □ Assessing parent knowledge, experience in providing discipline and consequences.
- Setting up rules.
  - □ Consistent across caregivers.
  - □ Importance to parent and adolescent functioning.
  - □ Able to assess compliance.
- Determining consequences.
  - □ Consistent across caregivers.
  - □ Practical and enforceable.
  - □ Reasonable.
  - □ Timely.
  - □ Types of consequences.
    - Allow natural consequences.
    - Remove or modify privileges: curfew, outings, event attendance, access to electronics/Internet/social media, allowance.
    - Pay restitution: extra chores, allowance fines.
    - Remove parental "favors": rides, laundry.
- Implementing rules and consequences.
  - □ Inform the adolescent.
  - □ The role of negotiation.
  - □ Handling postrule violation disputes.
- Role plays.
- Homework.
- Parent–adolescent home conference to review rules and consequences (may be done as part of parent–adolescent negotiation).
- Parent to keep monitoring and tracking log.

Debrief: Review of the Past Week, Interim Concerns, and Homework

The most common problem involved in establishing rules and consequences is the level of adolescent cooperation. In reviewing homework, the clinician should query about the level of adolescent resistance and how this was handled by the parent(s). Parents should report the results of rule compliance and violation and the reciprocal effects of parent–adolescent communication with rule compliance and violation.

Introducing Discipline and Negative Consequences

Many consider "discipline" to be synonymous with punishment rather than the broader notion of discipline as methods of modeling character and of teaching self-control and acceptable behavior, usually through the use of rules. Reviewing existing rules and establishing new rules is another essential task of PMT. Last week's homework asked parents to hold a conference with the adolescent to review monitoring and tracking rules. Clinicians should ask parents about their current household rules, the adolescent's response to the rules, and the parents' response to the adolescent's response. Based on these responses, the clinician and parents should assess the effectiveness of current rules.

Discipline extends beyond rule making. In most cases, adolescents with SUDs are not compliant with many household rules. This is usually because the consequences of rule violations are inadequate or the consequences are not implemented consistently by parents. Parent–adolescent interaction often follows a coercive behavior cycle wherein repeated parental requests are followed by teen noncompliance. This interaction escalates until either the parent gives up or forces the adolescent to comply. The inconsistency of the consequences exacerbates poor adolescent compliance. In addition, positive reinforcement of compliance (i.e., rewards) may be inadequate to promote improved adolescent compliance.

This session involves two PMT skills: (1) household rule assessment and rule development, and (2) determination of consequences for rule violation. Session 4 will focus on determination of rewards for rule compliance. These skills are closely related and eventually come together in a contract between the parent and adolescent. Development of a contract may involve parent–adolescent negotiation, a topic covered in Chapter 8. These aspects of PMT, including household rules, may not be finalized until parent–adolescent negotiation and agreement about a contract take place.

Setting Up Rules

Before taking on the development of new rules and consequences, the parent(s) should present and critically appraise current rules. How are these rules working to further the goals and solve the identified problems? Parents should be able to assess the teen's compliance with the rules, and rules should be consistent across other caregivers. In some cases, the parent's opinion of what is unacceptable may seem too strict or developmentally inappropriate. For example, requiring a certain grade average rather than asking that all homework be completed and turned in or that the adolescent spend a minimum amount of time each day on his or her schoolwork may not be a reasonable strategy. Rules should focus on a process. For example, limits on an adolescent's activities in terms of who, when, and where may be the best long-term strategy rather than saying the adolescent cannot go out with his or her friends, period. Particularly when reviewing rules that seem untenable and/or unfair, the clinician should maintain his or her role as a referee of sorts and ask the parents if the rule and/or consequences are practical and fair. The parents, helped by the clinician, rate the pros and cons of each rule. Similar to using parent–adolescent negotiation to help set up rules, parent and adolescents should review their perception of the success or failure of the rules.

Parents ultimately decide whether or not to change the rules. As noted in the discussion of parent–adolescent problem-solving skills, negotiating rules, particularly consequences for rule violations and rewards for rule compliance, take the adolescent's view into account. The final rules fall to the parents to decide.

When determining what the rules will be, several areas address the obvious adolescent behaviors that support substance use and the development of SUDs.

1. Monitoring.
   - When the adolescent will be home; curfews.
   - Communication when away from home.
2. Home.
   - Compliance with parent requests.
   - Chores and household responsibilities.
3. School.
   - Homework.
   - Attendance.
   - Level of achievement—expected grades.
4. Communication (see Session 5: Communication Skills).
   - How family members are addressed.

Determining Consequences

In determining consequences for rule violations, parents must be in agreement. The consequences should be practical and enforceable, timely (i.e., delivered as soon after the violation as possible), and reasonable (no grounding for long periods of time). The qualities of effective consequences are listed in Table 7.3.

TABLE 7.3. Qualities of Effective Consequences for Undesired Behavior(s)

1. Consequences should be established prior to occurrence of undesired behavior(s).
   - Parents should anticipate and plan for misbehavior.
2. Immediacy of consequences.
   - Consequences should occur as soon as possible after the behavior.
3. Specificity of consequences.
   - Specific consequences should be applied to each undesired behavior; deal with each behavior one at a time.
4. Predictability of consequences.
   - Specific consequence(s) imposed each and every time undesired behavior occurs.
5. Consistency of consequences.
   - Across settings, over time, and between parents and other caregivers.
6. Establish incentive programs for appropriate behavior before consequences are established.

In the context of substance use, deviant peers, and other deviant social activities, parents should be careful not to deliver a consequence that would cause the adolescent to miss a prosocial activity such as a school trip or planned socialization with a clearly prosocial peer or peer group. The importance of these prosocial activities as an alternative to substance use and other deviant behaviors and peers adds an important consideration in identifying and delivering consequences to adolescents.

While the groundwork for rules is set in PMT, the parents should take what they have discussed to parent–adolescent problem solving, where a rule may be negotiated with adolescent input.

Implementing Rules and Consequences

Once a rule is finalized, it is written down by parents and copies are distributed to family members. Rule violations should result with immediate, as much as possible, execution of the specific consequence. On a regular basis—weekly or biweekly—the family should review rules and compliance.

Role Plays

The clinician takes the part of one parent in developing rules or consequences with one of the parents. The clinician expresses common objections to specific nominated rules. In the case of a single parent, the clinician acts as a coach.

Homework

Parents develop a preliminary list of rules and consequences.

Session 4: Use of Positive Reinforcement, Rewards, and Contingency Management

Session Outline

- Debrief: Review of the past week and relevant interim concerns; review of homework.
- Introducing positive reinforcers/rewards.
  - □ Rationale: The importance of positive reinforcement/rewards.
  - □ Assessing parent knowledge and experience in providing reinforcers/rewards.
- Identifying reinforcers and rewards.
- The use of positive statements.
- Token economy.
- Role plays. The clinician should demonstrate how to bring up the topics of rewards and consequences with the adolescent, particularly what should be on the list of rewards and consequences. The parents, assuming the role of the adolescent, should both express how they think their teen would act when asked for their ideas about rewards and consequences and comment upon parental ideas.
- Homework.
  - □ Parent to keep monitoring and tracking log.
  - □ Plan family outing.

Debrief: Review of the Past Week, Interim Concerns, Homework

Review of this homework assignment may take up an entire session as the clinician reviews the preliminary rules with parents.

Introducing Positive Reinforcers/Rewards

Behavior change is facilitated by incentives (rewards and reinforcers) as well as disincentives (negative consequences, "punishments"). Behavior change is increased when reinforcers are available. Positive reinforcement is important not only for compliance with household rules but for any positive, prosocial behavior. Youth need lots of praise, attention, recognition, reward, support, and encouragement to develop prosocial behaviors. Adolescents also need expressions of warmth and caring from adults.

Contingency management refers to the delivery of rewards and positive reinforcers when good or desired behavior occurs (e.g., school attendance, compliance with household rules and parental requests) and consequences when undesired behavior occurs: If this happens . . . then the adolescent gets. . . . For an effective behavior plan, parents, with the assistance of the teen, need to identify a broad list of reinforcers (see Table 7.4). The removal of many positive reinforcers (e.g., cell phone or video game use) constitutes a consequence of undesired behavior as well.

Ask parents if they have had any experience in providing reinforcers and consequences.

Identifying Reinforcers and Rewards

Contingency management plans work well only if the adolescent knows the rules, consequences, and rewards beforehand. From a comprehensive list of reinforcers, the parent and the adolescent are to edit the items at home, with parents determining the final list. Each item must meet the following four criteria: (1) It does not contribute to irresponsible behavior, (2) it is nonessential, (3) the parent is willing and able to withhold the privilege if it's not earned, and (4) it's reasonable, given the context in which the youth and parent live (e.g., it's not too expensive). Parents must be able to monitor the target behavior in order to determine whether a reward (or consequence) is to be given. If the rewards are tied to specific behavior, then providing the designated reward is simple.

The Use of Positive Statements

Although I focus on tangible material goods, services, and privileges, other important positive reinforcers are social (e.g., hugs, praise, listening, attention, and spending time together). Reinforcers should be

TABLE 7.4. Potential Rewards and Other Reinforcers

■ Transportation	■ Curfew
■ Driving practice	■ Have a friend visit
■ Car privileges	■ Invite friend to sleepover
■ TV use	■ Nondrug, nonalcohol party or get-together
■ Trips with family and friends	
■ Meals out	■ Visit a friend's house
■ Favorite meal at home	■ Own phone or upgrade
■ One-on-one time with Dad or Mom	■ Movie tickets
■ Computer or other electronic equipment	■ Concert tickets
	■ Own room or sports equipment
■ Stuff for room (e.g., music equipment)	■ Laundry

individualized and based on the desires of the adolescent or what he or she is motivated to seek (positive) or avoid (negative).

Token Economy

Alternative contingency management programs involve a token economy where the contract clearly outlines what the youth can earn in points in return for adopting specific, prosocial behaviors or have points deducted for specific negative behaviors. Specific point deductions are made for specific undesired behaviors. The adolescent may receive "base points" at the beginning of each week. The contracting system may use escalating reinforcers in cases where there are no point deductions (no undesirable behaviors) in a given period (e.g., 1 week). For example, when a week (or month) has no point deductions, points may double for the following week (or month). The points are reset to the original level when there is a deduction or a recurrence of undesired behavior. Similarly, "bonus points" may be given when the teen achieves a specific number of points within a specific period of time or as a spontaneous reward in the event of a particularly positive behavior that is not covered in the contract. Parents should develop a way to monitor the point totals in the case of a token economy or through a list of behaviors with contingency rewards and punishments when a token economy is not used.

Role Plays

- *Practice positive statements.* The clinician sets a scenario in which the adolescent does something well. The parent is expected to respond in an unequivocally positive manner that is reinforcing.
- *List of reinforcers.* The clinician works with parents to develop a list of reinforcers for the adolescent's positive behavior.

Homework

Parents are asked to develop a comprehensive list of reinforcers to match with rule compliance. Remember, reinforcers should immediately follow the behavior. Therefore, it is essential to frequently review the results. Contingency management is an important element of PMT.

Session 5: Communication Skills

Session Outline

- Debrief: Review of past week and relevant interim concerns; review of homework.

- Introducing communication.
  - ▢ Rationale: The importance of positive communication.
  - ▢ Assessing parent knowledge, experience in communicating.
  - ▢ Rules of good communication.
- Modeling and role plays.
- Homework.

Debrief: Review Past Week, Interim Concerns, Homework

The list of reinforcers is reviewed. The clinician actively assists parents if they have difficulty coming up with ideas and advises on practical implementation.

Introducing Communication

Often, family therapy does not work unless there is satisfactory communication between parents and adolescents. Before teens and their parent(s) can negotiate, they need to be able to talk with one another in a productive, civil manner. Unfortunately, parent–adolescent relations are not always on the best terms in many of these cases. Teaching parents (and adolescents) a combination of improved communication, positive statements, and positive reinforcers will serve to improve the parent–adolescent relationship in the next phase of the therapy.

Several common communication-related problems are common in these families as listed in Table 7.5). They often have little, if any, communication, much less positive communication.

TABLE 7.5. Common Communication Problems

- Accusing, blaming
- Putting down, shaming
- Interrupting
- Lecturing, preaching, moralizing
- Commanding, ordering
- Threatening
- Talking through a third person
- Talking in a sarcastic tone
- Monopolizing the conversation
- Mind reading
- Dwelling on the past
- Getting off topic
- Psychologizing
- Failing to make eye contact
- Fidgeting, restlessness while others are talking
- Not responding

PARENT: You are making our lives crazy. You've screwed up our lives. You have been a bad kid since the first grade. You need to get your act together.

ADOLESCENT: I know you don't like me. As soon as I can, I am going to leave. . . . You won't let me get my driver's license.

PARENT: Watch it, buster! You are going to stay right here and listen to us. You need. . . .

ADOLESCENT: I don't need to do anything. I don't need to listen to you. You do not care about me.

Rules of Good Communication

There are a number of elements of good communication (see Table 7.6). The most important one is listening and allowing others a chance to express themselves without interruption by taking turns talking. Rather than "you" statements that convey a sense of fact, "I" statements are used to indicate that this is the thought of the person making the remark. For example, instead of "You are killing us," a parent could say, "I feel so badly about what is happening in your life" or "I think you are making poor decisions" rather than "You are wasting your life." Similarly, the feelings of others should be acknowledged ("I know you are angry at me"; "I know you do not like coming to treatment"). Controlling one's affect is also important, as most do not wish to listen to angry voices or harsh content. Swearing or vulgar or other disrespectful statements turn others off, and they stop listening or they respond in kind.

Feedback about behavior is always important. Parent(s) need to understand the distinction between a "concern" and "criticism" (here

---

TABLE 7.6. Rules for Communication

- When another is speaking, listen.
- One person speaks at a time; take turns.
- Use "I" statements.
- Acknowledge others' feelings.
- Restate what you just heard to check that you understand correctly.
- Do not swear or use vulgar language.
- Make no disrespectful comments to each other.
- Use positive statements about others: compliment sincerely, specifically, and immediately whenever appropriate.

framed negatively). Both the adolescent and parents should be able to express a concern describing how each feels about a specific issue or situation as opposed to making a "criticism" that is usually very general and expresses blame.

Criticism	*Concern*
"You *always* yell at me about my friends."	"I did not like it when you left last night without doing your chores."
"You don't trust me."	"I want to make some decisions on my own."
"You never do your homework."	"I am concerned about your failing grades and that maybe you will not finish school."

To communicate effectively with one another, parents and adolescents need to use good communication skills. Effective communication is necessary for implementation of PMT and parent–adolescent problem-solving skills.

Modeling and Role Plays

The clinician should have a good idea from previous contacts about the quality of communication between the adolescent and parent. The clinician should review elements of communication, model them, and then coach parents to practice by talking about less emotionally charged topics such as what types of meals family members would like or planning family outings. The clinician can coach members by pointing out poor communication practices, modeling examples of good communication, and reinforcing when parents begin to improve their communication styles and practices.

Clinicians should consider helping to expand opportunities for parent–adolescent discussion. Conversation should not only be about potentially contentious issues but should also include how the teen is doing—in school, with peers, romantic interests, and other concerns. The clinician should suggest venues for discussion such as family suppers, car trips, vacations, shopping, and even "dates" to attend events of common interest. Parents should be cautioned not to use these opportunities for lecturing, critical comments, or even any uninvited advice. The parents should listen, which serves to model and prompt similar behavior from the adolescent.

Parents should learn to compliment their teen as much as possible, saying something positive about his or her behavior or even the way the teen is phrasing his or her comments (if appropriate). Parents should praise the behavior and show appreciation by saying "thank you" whenever possible. For optimal effect, statement(s) should be *sincere, specific,* and *immediate* (i.e., expressed as soon as possible after the behavior). To avoid communication errors with their adolescents, parents may find it useful to provide feedback to each other about their mastery of these communication principles and techniques.

One valuable role play is for the clinician to play the role of the adolescent, demonstrating both positive and negative communication styles. Parents should attempt to respond using the guidelines for communication.

Homework

Ask the parents to arrange a situation in which conversation with the adolescent is likely (e.g., supper, family outing).

Session 6: Developing Contracts

Session Outline

- Debrief: Review of past week and relevant interim concerns; review of homework.
- Introducing developing contracts.
  - Rationale: The importance of contracts and positive communication.
  - Assessing parent knowledge, experience in providing reinforcers/ rewards and developing contracts with their adolescent or other children.
  - Introducing parent–adolescent problem solving.
  - Modeling and role plays. The clinician demonstrates the negotiation and contracting process with the parents, with the clinician initially taking the role of the parent and the parent(s) the role of the adolescent. Next, the parents assume their role as parents and the clinician becomes the adolescent.
  - Homework.
  - Parents develop a hierarchy (in order of importance) of issues for contracting.
  - Parents develop a comprehensive list of rules, consequences, and reinforcers.

Debrief: Review of the Past Week, Interim Concerns, Homework

INTRODUCING DEVELOPING CONTRACTS

Developing a contingency management plan involves putting consequences and reinforcers together. Then in the parent–adolescent problem-solving phase, a contract will be developed with the assistance of the adolescent. The contract details parental rules and expectations and the consequences and rewards for meeting or not meeting these rules. This session also prepares the parents for the parent–adolescent problem-solving phase.

RATIONALE

As suggested in earlier sessions, optimal behavioral management of the adolescent requires a balance of rewards and punishments or positive and negative contingencies when positive or negative behaviors are displayed. In other words, if there are consistent contingencies, a parent should see more or less of a behavior. For example, if the teen violates the family curfew rule, removing privileges should reduce subsequent violations. If the absence of rule violations is rewarded with an expansion of privileges, more positive behaviors can be expected.

CONTINGENCY CONTRACTS

When the behaviors, rewards, and consequences are agreed upon, they are written up and signed by both parents and adolescent. Written into the contract should be a procedure for modifying the contract after a specific period of time, for example, 2–3 months. I advocate specifying contingencies for attendance and compliance in a treatment program such as the recovery skills program described in Chapter 5 and parent and adolescent problem solving, described in Chapter 8. Although a program may provide motivational incentives, parents may further reinforce the effects of these incentives by providing additional rewards for negative drug tests and compliance with treatment.

Orientation to Parent–Adolescent Problem Solving

Results in setting up rules, obtaining consequences, or solving similar parent–adolescent issues are best when the adolescent feels he or she has a say. This is the basis for parent–adolescent problem solving where the adolescent joins parents in the discussion and negotiation of rules and consequences, and the development of contingency contracts. Much of

PMT is preparation for parent–adolescent problem solving. By preparing parents and adolescents separately, the parent–adolescent problem-solving session(s) often go more smoothly as each knows what to expect.

Parent management training and adolescent recovery skills training address skills deficits in parents and teenagers, respectively. At the conclusion of each of these elements, the clinician has oriented and prepared the parents and the adolescents for the family-based portion of our three-part intervention. They should now be ready to meet to negotiate contracts. This happens in the next phase of the behavioral family therapy model, parent–adolescent problem solving (see Chapter 8).

SUMMARY

Family-based interventions are among the best supported and most commonly used interventions for adolescents with SUDs. Although specific family-based interventions may vary in terms of theoretical emphasis and actual components, I have identified several salient elements, including the need to engage both parent(s) and teen; emphasize successful communication practices between parents and adolescents; improve parental skills in monitoring and supervising the adolescent; develop a system of appropriate rewards and consequences through the mutual contribution of parent and teen; and finally, develop family problem-solving skills to tackle both present and future problems.

Chapter Eight

Parent–Adolescent Problem Solving

The next phase of behavioral family-based therapy is family problem solving, which includes parent–adolescent negotiation. Parent–adolescent problem solving (PAPS) training is designed to improve communication between parents and their adolescent and to decrease the frequency and intensity of behavior problems in adolescents. This therapy model is a synthesis and elaboration of communications training (e.g., Goldstein, Sprifkin, Gershaw, & Klein, 1980) behavioral family therapy (e.g., Patterson & Forgatch, 1987), and problem-solving training (e.g., Robin & Foster, 1989).

PAPS training involves teaching parents and teenagers to negotiate how specific behavioral problems will be handled (e.g., noncompliance, arguing, poor schoolwork, curfews). It includes consequences for rule violation and reinforcers for compliance. In the areas that may be open for negotiation, the objective is to arrive at a "win–win" agreement such that both parents and teenagers gain something from the negotiated solution to a problem. Examples of areas for negotiation include how many times a week and when the adolescent may go out with friends, curfew times, allowance, specific times for homework, and chores,

The explicit goal of PAPS training is to teach parents and teenagers to write contracts that reflect compromises in areas of disagreement. This goal is achieved through the promotion of developmentally appropriate communication, problem solving, and personal responsibility. Achieving these goals depends on several skills, including keeping focused; using listening and empathy skills; taking personal responsibility for actions or feelings; stating problems specifically; and using compromise to resolve disagreements. Many parents and most teenagers are deficient in one or more of these skill areas. These deficits are serious impediments to effective communication and problem resolution. This is why I recommend communication skills training for parents in PMT and adolescents in the recovery skills program before beginning PAPS training.

The modest level of discussion of the adolescent's substance use in this family therapy model may surprise some. However, there is an explicit acknowledgment of substance use as a problem and as a target of treatment. Also explicit is that parents will not accept substance use by the adolescent. In addition, the CBT recovery skills described in Chapter 6 focus on the adolescent's substance use, and we recommend that teens learn these skills before, or concurrently with, family therapy. Family behavioral therapy focuses on parental behaviors and parent–adolescent interactions that promote adolescent substance use behaviors.

PARENT–ADOLESCENT NEGOTIATION

PAPS training involves teaching parents and teenagers to negotiate agreements about specific behavioral problems such as noncompliance with parents, arguing, failure to complete homework assignments, and failure to come home on time. While the term "negotiation" implies equal contribution by parents and adolescents, not all issues are negotiable. Parents retain veto power in areas they deem inappropriate for compromise, such as staying out all night or alcohol use in the home. The clinician needs to support the areas that parents see as non-negotiable. Areas that are open for negotiation include hair color and time to be home at night. For these, the objective is to arrive at a compromise agreement such that both parents and teenagers gain something from the negotiated solution. This procedure encourages adolescent autonomy and responsibility and is designed to improve communication and trust between parents and teenagers.

Before parents and teenagers meet to negotiate contracts, skill deficits, including communication, can be addressed by providing skill building. Preceding PAPS training, both recovery skills building and parent management training allow a more successful PAPS training experience for adolescent and parent alike. Adolescents attain communication skills such as making an appropriate complaint, accepting a limit set by others, knowing how to listen to others, recognizing the feelings of others, and learning how to negotiate (see Goldstein et al., 1980). Parents learn operant behavior theory, behavior analysis, how to make effective requests, how to set up a behavior change program, and how to recognize the

unique needs of adolescents with the cognitive and behavioral characteristics associated with the SUDs. While adolescent and parent skills building should usually precede PAPS training, a more experienced clinician
may combine each of these therapeutic approaches by alternatively seeing
families together and separately.

Session Structure

During the parent–adolescent negotiation phase, the parent and adolescent meet approximately once a week (45–60 minutes) for about 4 weeks.
The structure of PAPS training sessions varies, depending on the timing of the session relative to other components of the therapy such as
adolescent skills training and PMT, the nature of the issues presented by
the family, and the pace of developing problem-solving skills. Generally
speaking, each session begins with a review of homework and current concerns of parents and adolescents. As long as there are unresolved issues,
the parent will alternate with the teenager in presenting an issue. They
then deal with that one issue until they create a negotiated agreement
with a mutually satisfactory solution to the issue. Finally, when agreement
is reached on each of the presented issues, the results are written down in
the form of a contract, signed by parents and adolescent. Contracts may
vary in complexity, but at the very least they should be written and include
a reevaluation date, which may be as soon as the next PAPS training session. Adolescents and parents are prompted prior to therapy sessions to
come prepared with an issue for problem solving. During the sessions,
the clinician should encourage parents and teenagers to communicate
effectively, stay on task, and develop a written agreement about a specific
behavioral issue.

The structure of the sessions (both physical and interpersonal) should
promote direct interactions between parent and teenager. For example,
parents and teenagers should face each other (preferably across a table),
and the clinician should gradually move away from the table so that he or
she is in the family's peripheral vision rather than in their line of sight.

The clinician should spend the last 5–10 minutes of each session
reviewing adherence to each of the PAPS guidelines (Figure 8.1). The
guidelines should be reviewed individually, and each family member
should be asked for his or her opinion on how well that member performed. Positive comments about others should be strongly praised.
Many families will have considerable difficulties with the process and will
need extensive direction and skill development training (e.g., role-playing
situations). Clinicians should remind families that are having difficulties
that it takes time to develop the skills and *that it may help to focus on one
communication principle at a time.* It may also be helpful to ask that parents

1. Find the proper time and place to negotiate. Everyone must be calm, yet interested. Negotiation should not be undertaken when family members are extremely angry or when a problem seems so remote that it is not meaningful. Sit around a table or in upright chairs.

2. Start by stating an issue to negotiate. Parents identify an issue, and the adolescent identifies an issue (in random order). Parents state what is non-negotiable.

3. The essence of negotiation is compromise. Neither the parent nor the adolescent will get exactly what they want.

4. The parent and adolescent should state the best possible and the least acceptable solution for each issue to be negotiated.

5. State clearly what you want from each other, and don't bluff hoping for a better outcome. Don't assume that you know what will be said.

6. There are consequences for not negotiating. For an adolescent, failing to negotiate will likely be total parental control of decisions affecting the adolescent.

7. Use your communication skills:

   a. Take responsibility for your feelings and issues. Start sentences with "I." Avoid "you" statements.

   b. Use words that are not emotionally charged (e.g., "I would like you to be home at 4:00 P.M.," not "Be home at 4:00 P.M. or you're in big trouble").

   c. Practice what you are going to say before the session so that you can talk without too much emotion.

   d. Restate or paraphrase what was just said to check that you understood correctly—for example, "Did I just hear you say that you did not go to school today?" Make sure that parents and adolescent perceive the situation in the same way.

8. Negotiate in good faith. Don't reserve decisions until after the session and say to yourself, "I don't have to do what I said I would because I didn't really want to and I just said that because we were meeting."

(continued)

FIGURE 8.1. Guidelines for negotiating.

9. Talk in specifics, not generalities (e.g., "Come home at 5:00," not "Take responsibility for yourself"). Focus on one specific issue at a time.

10. Talk in the present and the future, not the past. Do not repeatedly discuss a past situation. Discuss what you can do to change the situation in the future.

11. Parents must not dictate to their adolescent. The adolescent must not demand privileges from the parents. Rather, they should discuss and compromise.

13. If anger occurs, take a time-out from the conversation until you are in control of yourself. If your attention drifts, take a short break and attempt to focus again.

14. Acknowledge each other's feelings and apologize when you are wrong.

15. Agree when you can. If you can agree on one small point, do so. Do not assume that you must agree on everything you want from each other.

16. If either parent or teen doesn't like what the other presents as a solution to a problem, then that person has an obligation to present an alternate solution.

17. Decide how any solution reached will be monitored. For example, if a parent is not home when the adolescent arrives, how will that parent know the teen arrived on time?

18. Don't ask for a commitment until the end of the session.

19. Write down what you have decided.

20. The parents and adolescent should sign their names to show that they understand what they have negotiated. Neither parent nor adolescent can change the written decisions without a negotiation session, except in an emergency. The family should define "emergency."

FIGURE 8.1. *(continued)*

and teenagers *not* try to use the problem-solving process outside of the PAPS training sessions until after they have successfully negotiated and positively evaluated a few contracts with the aid of a PAPS training clinician. All family members should be praised for successive approximations toward mastering each skill.

The Role of the Clinician

During these sessions, the clinician should take a "coaching" approach. This means, for example, that the family should be encouraged to generate and evaluate their own solutions and to speak directly to each other as opposed to or through the clinician. The primary challenge to the PAPS training clinician will be to keep the family working at an efficient pace and avoiding protracted or unnecessary conflict. The clinician will also monitor and prompt the correct use of communication skills learned in previous sessions. Video or audio recording of sessions is often useful in having the family evaluate their own skills. This clinician stance and concern with quickly arriving at an agreement is intended to promote creation of written contracts independent of clinician input and to maintain the adolescent's attention, motivation, and cooperation. Of course, different families and issues require varying amounts of clinician involvement. The clinician should be very active in reinforcing adherence to problem-solving guidelines, generalizing skills learned prior to the PAPS training session, and praising successive approximations toward the independent implementation of the PAPS training procedure.

As the name implies, the clinicians are expected to help parents and teenagers communicate with each other. As I previously suggested, separate adolescent skills training and PMT can be used as preliminary sessions to increase engagement and identify and understand specific issues that may generate overt conflict. The clinician should have the family's trust and be seen as an advocate for the interests of the adolescent and parents, respectively.

The Initial PAPS Training Session

The first session should begin by explaining the role of the PAPS training clinician to the family. Points to make include telling them the goal is for the parent(s) and teenager to negotiate independently such that each party has an issue resolved and the resolution recorded in specific terms in writing. Accordingly, the family will be asked to speak to each other rather than to or through the clinician and will be expected to try to come up with their own solutions before the PAPS training clinician will offer any suggestions. The clinician's main responsibility is to give feedback about how the family is following the guidelines and to help them keep on task and on time.

Reviewing and Practicing the Negotiation Guidelines

Each family member should be provided with his or her own copy of the problem-solving worksheet (Figure 8.2) as well as the guidelines for negotiating (Figure 8.1). The clinician should explain that adolescent and parents alternate in choosing issues and then review each of the guidelines for communication and problem solving. The PAPS training process is summarized in Table 8.1.

1. What is my problem?

2. What is my goal?

3. What are some possible solutions?

4. How well would each possible solution work?

5. Pick the best solution and try it.

6. Did I pick the right one?

FIGURE 8.2. Problem-solving worksheet.

TABLE 8.1. The Parent–Adolescent Problem-Solving Process

1. Adolescent or parent selects an issue. The issue is defined and written down in plain language.
2. Whoever brought up the issue suggests a solution.
3. The second party should restate the proposed solution, ask for clarification of the proposal, and either accept it or suggest another possible solution.
4. The clinician may encourage trading and compromise and should monitor communication and correct when necessary.
5. Alternative solutions continue to be proposed by the two sides alternating until there is mutual agreement to a current proposed solution. When agreement is reached, a contract is written and signed by all parties, including the clinician.
6. This process is repeated with the next issue.
7. The family should not use the parent–adolescent problem-solving process outside sessions until told to do so (after experience negotiating several contracts within sessions).
8. The family is sent home to fulfill and monitor existing contracts.

Each of the guidelines for negotiating (Figure 8.1) is discussed next. The clinician should then model and direct role plays covering the 20 problem-solving guidelines. These models and role plays should begin during the first session and should be completed about halfway through the second session. The clinician should alternately take the role of parent and adolescent.

The teen and his or her parents have two options to arrive at a list of potential solutions to each problem or issue. The first option consists of one party offering a proposed solution to the problem, advocating for that solution, with the other party either accepting that solution or presenting an alternative. Solutions are exchanged until a compromise or impasse is reached—a true negotiation. The alternative option, brainstorming, involves the adolescent and parents together generating a list of potential solutions without pausing to critically evaluate each one. Brainstorming is reserved for use in the event of an impasse or for clinician or family preference because, in my clinical experience, families take an inordinately long time to resolve problems using this option.

ROLE PLAY

The clinician chooses a relatively benign issue (e.g., eating together on a specific night, minor chore[s]), and each party, in turn, provides potential solutions or alternatives until a final solution is agreed upon. The clinician repeats the issue and solution and writes the solution down.

Choosing an Issue for Consideration

After this brief orientation and role play is completed, the clinician should randomly pick which party (the parent or teenager) will go first in selecting an issue. This is usually accomplished by having the clinician, or a family member, draw from an envelope or similar container a slip of paper that has "parent" or "teenager" written on it. The first party chosen should state their issue, and the second party replies with an alternative or agrees to the previously stated solution. I recommend advising the family to start with an easier issue first, not the most contentious one. As the family becomes more experienced with PAPS, they can work on more difficult, emotionally charged issues.

It is important to begin the problem-solving process with a clear and specific written definition of the issue. Although this step may seem tedious, it is crucial to effective communication and successful contracting. In many instances, defining the issue may be the most time-consuming step of the problem-solving process. Defining the issue usually begins by having one party state and the other restate the issue. Parents and teenagers should discuss the definition and solutions until the statements and restatements are specific and agree with each other. Agreement should be praised and written down on the problem-solving worksheet (Figure 8.2). The clinician should also be aware that this is a good time to role-model, prompt, or reward the use of reframing. For example, when an adolescent states that he or she does not want to have a curfew, parents reframe the issue as what time the curfew should be.

Parents and teenagers are under no obligation to negotiate on any issue. Indeed, an important consideration in the PAPS training process is that parents have the ultimate responsibility for their adolescents and can define any issue (usually a limit) as non-negotiable. For example, it is perfectly acceptable for a parent to state that issues related to school attendance or drug use (either therapeutic or illicit) are not open for negotiation and compromise. These issues are often identified earlier during PMT training, so that the parent(s) are prepared, having discussed this matter and determined what issues are negotiable and what issues are not. This "fail-safe" procedure is very important to parents, who often express concerns that the PAPS process will undermine their authority and require them to accept what is, in their opinion, completely unacceptable behavior. In some cases, however, the parents' opinion of what is unacceptable may seem too strict or developmentally inappropriate. For instance, a parent may not allow his or her adolescent to watch certain television programs, browse the Internet, or go on dates. Parents' decisions to make an issue non-negotiable should not be challenged in the first session. If the clinician disagrees with a parental limit, this should have been discussed with them in PMT training (see Session 3 in Chapter 7). If the parents persist in defining the issue as non-negotiable, the clinician must respect this decision but should point out the natural consequences. For example, they can be reminded that not allowing a teenager to date may interfere with the development of age-appropriate relationships and social skills.

Example of Determining a Curfew

CLINICIAN: Emma [the adolescent] goes first.

ADOLESCENT: I want to talk about curfew. I don't think I should have one, but I think midnight on weekdays and 2:00 A.M. on weekends should be okay. I know my friends can stay out that late. Some don't even have any curfews.

PARENT: This is a bit late. You have to get up the next morning on weekdays—so I think 10:00 P.M.

ADOLESCENT: Some activities don't start until 8:00 P.M.—I can't get home by then. What about 10:00 P.M. except for activities.

PARENT: I am willing to consider up until 11 P.M. only when there is an activity—and you have to show me the schedule.

ADOLESCENT: I can live with that, but what about weekends—I can sleep later.

PARENT: Actually, your new job starts at 10:00 A.M. I think midnight is fine.

ADOLESCENT: OK.

CLINICIAN: Are there any other conditions that you would like to consider for the curfew issue?

Adolescents may respond very negatively to having a parent define an issue as non-negotiable. In most instances, the parent's definition of an issue as non-negotiable should be supported by the clinician, although teenagers should be encouraged to acknowledge their parents' feelings even if they do not agree. In these instances, the teenager should be reminded of the opportunities for improving his or her negotiating position by earning trust, and the possibility later of easing the limit through compliance. Teenagers may also be reminded that although the specific issue might remain firm and non-negotiable, they could improve the status of their "emotional bank account" by accepting a specific non-negotiable limit.

Teenagers do not have the authority to define an issue as non-negotiable, but they can opt out of discussion of a parent-defined issue. In these instances, the parents should be asked if they accept the teenager's decision not to negotiate on the issue. If the parent insists on discussing the issue, the teenager cannot, and should not, be forced to negotiate. However, teenagers who refuse to discuss the issue are expected to accept any decision made by their parents as a consequence of not negotiating. The clinician should remind the teenager that refusing to negotiate takes away the opportunity to address their parents as a psychological equal. The natural consequence of this decision is that the relationship may revert back to the parent–adolescent ("one-up, one-down") stance. In other words, teenagers who do not negotiate must accept that parents make decisions independent of the teenager's input.

ADOLESCENT: I should not have to have urine tests [drug screens]! I have been going to school. I have not gotten into trouble.

PARENT: Larry, I'm afraid right now that is non-negotiable. We appreciate that you have been doing better, and we have demonstrated that appreciation by letting you go out of the house more and see some of your friends. But the program requires the drug screens. We have been rewarding your negative screens. I know that, eventually, they will stop the screens.

Negotiating

Once the issue is agreed upon and written in specific language, the clinician should prompt the person who brought up the issue to propose a solution. The second party should restate the proposed solution, ask for clarification of the proposal, and either accept the proposal or suggest an alternative. Generally, the negotiation takes the form of considering the pros and cons and possible outcomes for each solution offered using basic problem-solving steps. Adolescents will have learned these steps in their recovery skills sessions, but clinicians may find it useful to review the basic problem-solving principles with parents: (1) define and formulate the problem, (2) generate multiple possible solutions, (3) evaluate the pros and cons of each solution and choose one, and (4) evaluate whether the solution worked. However, the PAPS technique modifies the problem-solving technique; instead of step 2, the generation of multiple possible solutions, the adolescents have responsibility for suggesting an alternative if they cannot accept the solution offered by the parents. In this manner, the adolescent is able to contribute and have more control over the situation. The PAPS training clinicians should be familiar with these social skills learned in adolescent recovery skills training and be prepared to prompt or praise the adolescent for use of these skills.

The clinician should be especially attentive to encouraging a give-and-take (trading and compromise) approach. Beware of discussions that degenerate into what the parents will provide materially if the adolescent does what the parents want. For example, rather than allowing the parents to pay the adolescent money for cleaning his or her bedroom, they could allow a later curfew if the room passes weekly inspection. It is important to emphasize that the goal in this process is to achieve a "win–win" situation in which both persons may not get exactly what they want, but they will both get something out of the deal. This is contrasted with a "win–lose" situation in which one person does all of the giving and the other does all of the taking.

CLINICIAN: I see that the parents have chosen doing homework as the next issue to resolve.

ADOLESCENT: I am not sure I want to talk about school.

CLINICIAN: I want to remind you that we have already discussed several of your issues—curfew, attending school activities, and bedtime. It's your parents' turn.

PARENT: Yes, we are concerned about Bobby getting his homework done. He may fail this semester due to uncompleted homework.

ADOLESCENT: OK.

CLINICIAN: So let's take turns and throw out some solutions—Bobby, you go first.

ADOLESCENT: I promise to do homework; they just need to trust me.

PARENT: That's the way it is now . . . and it's not working!

CLINICIAN: Parents, your turn, offer a solution.

PARENTS: I think one of us should supervise his homework.

ADOLESCENT: You are not always around when I do my homework—you can check it before I go to school.

PARENT: Well, we are not always around then either. How about Bobby completing his homework right after school, before he does anything else.

CLINICIAN: How would you check to make sure it is done and handed in?

PARENT: The school has a homework website—we can check it off using that.

CLINICIAN: Bobby, what do you think?

ADOLESCENT: I don't need my homework checked.

CLINICIAN: I recall your parents accepting a negotiated curfew—later than they wanted.

ADOLESCENT: I guess I can live with it.

CLINICIAN: What happens if homework is *not* completed?

PARENT: He can't go out that evening or the next day. If he does not make it up, then he cannot go out for 2 weeks.

ADOLESCENT: That's way too much. How about just the next weekend?

PARENTS: OK.

ADOLESCENT: But what do I get if I do my homework?

CLINICIAN: Can you offer a reinforcer for a period of successful homework completion?

PARENT: How about for each night of homework completion, you get an extra 30 minutes of screen time?

ADOLESCENT: Let's write this down!

In the give-and-take exchange, it is sometimes possible to create a contract that simultaneously addresses the parent's and teenager's issues. For example, if the parent's issue is homework completion and the teenager's issue is curfew, then making a later curfew contingent on homework completion resolves both issues in one contract. This is an ideal situation that may or may not occur for some families. It is mentioned here to point out that the clinician is not obligated to negotiate issues separately. In fact, the opposite is desired but is not always possible.

The clinician will find that there is a great deal to cover in the time allotted for the 45- to 60-minute problem-solving sessions. Although longer sessions may proceed at a more relaxed pace, several difficulties might arise with longer sessions. The chief concern is that longer sessions will be less generalizable than shorter sessions. More specifically, families are probably more likely to negotiate an issue if it only takes 10–15 minutes as opposed to 30 minutes or longer. Another concern is that longer sessions will be less focused and run a greater risk of nonproductive conflict. Thus, clinicians should be very attentive to the duration as well as to the quality of the PAPS negotiation. The efficiency of PAPS is greatly facilitated by having specific agreed-upon issues, keeping on task, and avoiding dwelling on the past. In addition, after families get the hang of it, specific issues can be assigned as homework. Remember, the ultimate goal is for the family to be able to negotiate and problem solve without the clinician.

Subsequent Sessions

I generally expect a minimum of three to four problem-solving sessions. After the second session, subsequent sessions begin with an evaluation of the status of contracts that are in effect. This should include a discussion of compliance by both parties, the clarity of the contract, the feasibility of monitoring the contingencies, and the ability to provide rewards specified in the contract. Discussions of new issues or a general appraisal of the period between meetings should be postponed until the contracts have been reviewed. This allows the clinician and family to focus on the "real-life" application of the PAPS model, learn from mistakes, and bask in accomplishments. It is pointless to negotiate new contracts if the old ones are not working. Moreover, this review process stresses the importance of periodically reevaluating the contracts. If a contract has not yet been negotiated (i.e., they ran out of time before a written contract could be completed during the previous meeting), the session should begin where previous discussions left off. This stresses the importance of completing one contract discussion before moving on to the next. Depending on the family's skill level and the volatility of a particular issue, it may be possible to give the family a homework assignment to complete problem solving and begin the next session with a review of the new contract. In these cases, sessions may begin with a review of contracts negotiated at home.

After the first few PAPS sessions, the clinician should try to let the family negotiate the contracts as independently as possible. The family should successfully negotiate a contract with practically no input from the clinician before they are discharged from treatment. This may involve having a homework assignment to negotiate a contract or having the family negotiate a contract with the understanding that the clinician will say nothing until the contract is written and signed.

Dealing with Alcohol and Other Drug Use

Substance use by the adolescent should be non-negotiable. Much of the parent–adolescent negotiation discussed thus far has been centered on preventing the adolescent from participating in high-risk situations and behaviors and increasing prosocial behavior—for example, tracking what the adolescent does and setting up rules on where he or she can go and with whom. Parents should also want to increase the adolescent's participation in prosocial activities with prosocial peers and minimize the opportunities to use drugs or alcohol.

With regard to drug or alcohol use, parents need to determine the consequences of use—the consequences of a positive drug screen (or refusal to provide a sample) and positive reinforcement for compliance with a drug screen and a negative screen.

PARENT: I feel we should talk about Chuck's drinking.

ADOLESCENT: Hey, I have to get a curfew, be in school every day. How am I going to blow off steam? All my friends drink. Their parents don't mind.

PARENTS: Well, no drinking—or any other drug use—is going to be one of our rules.

ADOLESCENT: Another *rule*! What's in this for me?

CLINICIAN: I understand Chuck's point. Is there anything you can offer if he does not use alcohol or marijuana?

PARENT: I don't know what we can do.

CLINICIAN: Chuck, any ideas?

ADOLESCENT: Buy me a car if I don't use.

CLINICIAN: I suspect your parents will feel that a car is a bit pricey.

ADOLESCENT: What about money—more allowance!

CLINICIAN: Well, you have already negotiated a resumption of your allowance, assuming you do the chores outlined in the contract you are making with your parents.

PARENT: How do we do that—reward him for no alcohol or marijuana use?

CLINICIAN: You could add a specific amount for each period of no use or negative urine drug screens or attendance at any treatment-related activities such as Chuck's school group, AA meetings. We just need a way of monitoring his compliance with these required activities.

ADOLESCENT: But what about a car?

CLINICIAN: Although a car is still probably out of reach for your parents, they could consider a bonus reward if you pass a certain period—say 3 or 6 months—of regular treatment attendance and negative drug screens.

ADOLESCENT: But what if I don't want to test my pee all the time?

PARENT: You're going to have to do the drug screens.

CLINICIAN: Doing the screens is the only way we can know for sure whether you are using or not. In order to get bonuses or other rewards—and keep your privileges—we need to be able to measure these behaviors.

PARENT: But how can we make him do the screens? He's given us trouble about this before.

CLINICIAN: We advise parents to consider that a refusal to screen has the same consequences as a positive urine screen. I know we have talked about your consequences for Chuck's having a positive test—the loss of specific privileges, grounding for a specific time. I know he's a gamer; loss of computer or cell phone time would be serious for Chuck. He agreed and even came up with many of these consequences himself.

PARENT: I like this—it gives us some structure.

CLINICIAN: Chuck, how do you feel?

ADOLESCENT: I guess it's OK. I still think I should get a car for all of this!

The clinician and parents should begin with less controversial issues to negotiate than substance use. As the adolescents see that they have *some* influence on the outcome, they often become more engaged with the model. More heated topics such as substance use become easier to undertake.

In the case of the pervasively resistant teen, the clinician and parent(s) should still proceed through the process. The clinician can attempt to take the adolescent's perspective and continue to attempt to elicit suggestions from the adolescent as to what issues to discuss, consequences for undesirable behavior, and rewards for desired behavior.

In the final session with a PAPS training clinician, the family is expected to review their progress, identify future areas of skill development, discuss their ability to negotiate contracts without having a clinician present, and consider appropriate follow-up services. Booster sessions can be scheduled throughout succeeding months, as needed, to reinforce skills.

Negotiating Contracts at Home

Families should be encouraged to continue using the PAPS process even after discharge from treatment. Home maintenance should include periodic (at least once a month) family discussions to review contracts. During these discussions, the parents should be encouraged to remember the four principles for working with adolescents that are taught during parent training: (1) think small, (2) be consistent, (3) nurture autonomy, and (4) think long-term. The PAPS training program is designed to anticipate problems and prevent unnecessary conflict in the future. It is not intended to be used as needed to diffuse crises.

The basic guidelines for home problem solving or negotiation are fairly simple and follow the procedures used with the clinician. The family should schedule meetings. They should sit facing each other across a table and have materials for writing a contract. Each party should state their issue to be discussed. The order of issues can be decided by a flip of a coin. The discussions should follow the PAPS guidelines as specified in Figure 8.2. The family should take a break if emotion is expressed inappropriately or if there is repeated noncompliance with requests by one party. Written contracts should be made for each issue, with a reevaluation date specified for every contract. At the end of the problem solving, the family should review adherence to the PAPS guidelines and adolescents should identify areas in which they can personally improve the PAPS process.

For all aspects of therapy for adolescents with SUDs and their families, booster sessions may be both needed and advisable. The format of the booster session is flexible, although the sessions will take on a primarily PAPS format. At each session, the clinician will review past and current contracts and problem-solving efforts. The clinician will reinforce positive progress or assist the family in identifying and dealing with impediments to successful contract negotiation, compliance, and results. The clinician may help the family renegotiate old contracts or develop new ones for emerging issues. The clinician will assess the adolescent's attainment of skills and may elect to use booster session time to refresh or reinforce skills through practice and review.

Troubleshooting

Resistance

Overt or covert resistance to behavioral family therapy activities on the part of either adolescent or parents makes progress difficult, although working without the adolescent is possible (see below). Use of MI techniques and "rolling with resistance," in particular, is the best strategy (see Chapter 2). Unreasonable beliefs and expectations commonly underlie resistance. The clinician deals with parental beliefs and expectations proactively through his or her initial explanation of adolescent development and reasonable expectations. The clinician always needs to acknowledge and be sympathetic to parental concerns.

RESISTANT PARENTS

Engagement and empathy are important in decreasing resistance and ambivalence. Resistance may be due to parents expecting the clinician to fix their teen. At the outset, the clinician should describe his or her expectations of treatment, which include (1) active parental involvement; and (2) resolving parent factors that hinder treatment, such as interparent communication and relationship issues. Parental SUDs and/or mental health issues are common occurrences, and resistance to treatment is likely. I like to reframe these problems as obstacles to helping their child. Parents might have greater motivation to address their own issues if that helps their child. Finally, parents may have a bias against some intervention modalities. Providing some level of choice may be necessary to get parents on board for treatment.

> PARENT 1: Why are we expected to come to treatment? It's Tom's problem.
>
> CLINICIAN: You did not expect to have to come to any treatment sessions? It's really not your problem at all.
>
> PARENT 1: It's not that; we could probably help, but what would my husband and I do at rehab?
>
> CLINICIAN: I know you really are concerned and want to help, but you are not sure how to help.
>
> PARENT 2: Yes, we're not sure, but I know we have to stop the fighting. I'm afraid I'm going to have a heart attack!
>
> CLINICIAN: So it's important to communicate better. That is an effort parents can help with.
>
> PARENTS: Yes, we think so, but Tom has to stop using.
>
> CLINICIAN: I agree; there are some things that Tom can do to help, but it is important for us to cover any area that might be contributing to his problems.

Adolescent Refusal to Participate

The adolescent's refusal to participate in PAPS is not an uncommon occurrence. Although the clinician should extend an open invitation to the adolescent to participate at any point in the treatment process, he or she should proceed with parents in the PMT and communication portions of the behavioral family therapy. With both the open invitation and the work with parents, clinician and parents create a program through which the adolescent receives positive reinforcement for eventual participation and the contingency management program. The clinician reassures parents that their unilateral efforts can have positive effects.

Poor and Malignant Communication

Despite meeting with parents and adolescents individually and later together to develop more positive communication skills, negative communication patterns may persist or be difficult to manage. There may be obscenities, and a physical altercation may ensue. The family may have difficulty being in the same room together, much less having a constructive discussion about contentious issues. In such cases, the clinician should consider several strategies: (1) starting parallel sessions with adolescent and parents separately; (2) intensive coaching on more effective communication with demonstrations, role plays, and even audio and video replays of sessions to allow for self-correction of communication errors; and (3) using scripts or written messages until each party can verbally communicate appropriately.

Clinicians should conduct one more parallel session to prepare each party—parent(s) and adolescent—for the parent–adolescent negotiation phase. During these separate sessions, the clinician introduces communication skills training, demonstrates skills, and coaches each party through role plays. Both in these separate sessions and later during communication skills training and negotiation phases, the clinician starts with more benign issues and, as the family demonstrates more communication competence, moves to the more contentious issues. Demonstration of improved communication skills as well as tolerance of parent or adolescent perceptions and constructive criticism is positively reinforced. Examples of poor, negative communication are rephrased in a more positive fashion. When the family demonstrates improvement, the clinician suggests a family outing during which the family members focus on and provide only positive statements about the behavior of other family members.

MODIFICATION OF PARENT–ADOLESCENT NEGOTIATION

This chapter describes a four-session protocol, which may be most appropriate and practical for an outpatient setting. The clinician may wish to modify the protocol in terms of the number of sessions and the skills emphasized. For example, in the context of a brief inpatient psychiatric hospitalization and fewer available sessions, the clinician may focus on rules for negotiation and setting up an agenda for negotiation while allowing less time for practice and role playing. For some families, the duration may need to be extended to allow for more practice, role playing, and coaching for individual family members.

The age of the adolescent may also suggest some modifications in the clinician's approach. Younger adolescents may need more coaching and direction for their participation. Using menus of topics for negotiation and more role-plays are examples of the need for increased structure in working with younger adolescents. The parent-generated topics for negotiation are often age related with general behavior concerns (e.g., curfew, school, peers) characteristic of younger teens, while more specific substance use behaviors (e.g., treatment attendance, urine drug screens) may increase with the age of the adolescent.

SUMMARY

Family-based interventions are among the best supported and most commonly used interventions for adolescents with substance use disorders. Although specific family-based interventions may vary in terms of the theoretical emphasis and actual components, I have identified several salient elements, including the need to engage both parent(s) and teen, emphasize successful communication practices between parents and adolescents, improve parental skills in monitoring and supervising the adolescent, develop a system of appropriate rewards and consequences through the mutual contribution of parent and teen, and finally, develop family problem-solving skills to tackle both present and future problems.

Chapter Nine

Integrated Treatment for Substance Use Disorders and Other Psychiatric Disorders

Coexisting emotional and behavioral problems are the rule rather than the exception for adolescents with SUDs. As discussed in Chapter 1, 82% of youth in treatment for SUDs have a non-SUD psychiatric diagnosis. Both externalizing disorders (ADHD, oppositional defiant disorder, and conduct disorder) and internalizing disorders (mood and anxiety disorders) have rates exceeding 40–50% of adolescents in treatment for SUDs. In this chapter, I discuss treatment approaches for coexisting psychiatric disorders and how these can be integrated into SUD treatment in youth. Among the risk factors for the development of SUDs in adolescents are a number of comorbid psychiatric disorders. "Comorbidity" refers to the coexistence of two or more diagnosable mental disorders and, in this case, two or more substance use disorders and mental illnesses, with each meeting DSM-5 criteria. For children and adolescents, "comorbidity" has been used interchangeably with the term "dual diagnosis," although in many cases there are more than two diagnoses. Although I emphasize disorders meeting full DSM criteria, one should still consider as a potential comorbidity and intervention target any problem that includes symptoms and results in impairment.

The most common comorbid psychiatric disorders among youth in addictions treatment include conduct (disorder) problems, oppositional defiant disorder, ADHD, mood disorders (e.g., depression), and trauma-related symptoms and disorders. Comorbid disorders are important in several respects (Kaminer, 2015). They are both markers for severity and potential targets for treatment. Among treated adolescents, comorbid psychopathology, particularly conduct problems and major depression, generally predicts early return to substance use. Co-occurring psychopathology also generally predicts a more persistent course of substance involvement over 1-year follow-up and likely over the adolescent's lifetime. For example, depression is one of the most robust predictors of relapse for adolescents. Comorbid psychopathology may precede, exacerbate, or follow the onset of heavy substance use. A review of adolescent community surveys found that the presence of childhood psychiatric disorders generally predicted earlier initiation of substance use and SUD onset, particularly when the childhood disorder was conduct disorder. While self-medication as a basis for the development and/or maintenance of SUDs is perhaps overstated, clearly any relief from depression, anxiety, anger, or adverse emotional states can be reinforcing and promote regular or increased substance use. Comorbidity has an influence on the development and persistence of SUDs and related behaviors. Clinicians should recognize the importance of identifying comorbid disorders in assessment and target them for intervention as part of a comprehensive and preferably integrated treatment plan.

For the most part, however, "dual treatment" has involved either serial or sequential treatment or parallel interventions in each of two separate systems. Adolescents with co-occurring disorders often fail to receive effective treatment. Although both mental health and substance use disorders are broadly considered psychiatric conditions and are contained in DSM-5, there has long been a divergence in how they are assessed and treated. Many of the obstacles to treatment for either psychiatric disorders or SUDs such as stigma, resistance, family stressors, or familial psychopathology are often compounded in cases of comorbidity.

CAN SUBSTANCE USE
AND PSYCHIATRIC TREATMENTS COEXIST?

The integration of treatment for SUDs and psychiatric disorders offers significant challenges (see Libby & Riggs, 2008). Traditional behavioral health treatment in this country revolves around separate and often disconnected systems of treatment for SUDs and other psychiatric disorders. Conceptualizations of illness and corresponding treatment philosophies have been profoundly different. In the past two to three decades, efforts toward development of dual-disorders programs have emerged, initially allowing those with both SUDs and psychiatric disorders to be treated in a single treatment environment where traditional modalities for each treatment are available. For example, in many programs, both 12-step approaches and medications, when appropriate, are provided to patients. More recently, to promote the concurrent treatment of SUDs and psychiatric disorders, researchers and clinicians have developed integrated approaches in which single modalities such as family therapy or CBT are modified to target problems across SUDs and psychiatric disorders. For example, family therapy targets improved adolescent–parent communication and parental monitoring, resulting in reduction in substance use as well as other disruptive behaviors. CBT can target substance use behaviors as well as depression, anxiety, problem solving, and anger control.

Despite the efforts of such agencies as the Substance Abuse and Mental Health Services Administration (SAMHSA) to promote a comprehensive approach to comorbidity assessment and intervention, information and training activities are relatively brief, lack follow-up and monitoring, and require supervision for optimal implementation by practitioners. Educational backgrounds, training experiences, and licensing requirements often vary widely between mental health and substance abuse treatment communities. Only recently have significant cross-training opportunities emerged, as well as incentives and resources for seeking them out once students have become practitioners. There are no widely accepted models for specialist certification in co-occurring disorders, and becoming dually certified or licensed in each system may be beyond the feasibility of most practitioners. As a result, few providers are sufficiently knowledgeable to treat co-occurring disorders.

Differences in training and philosophy have historically contributed to a lack of consensus on treatment planning, creating difficulties with coordination and collaboration across systems. Unfortunately, poor communication and coordination are also noted between behavioral health care systems and other child-serving agencies, such as education, child welfare, juvenile justice, and medical health care. This is especially problematic for youth with co-occurring disorders because of the multiple systems serving these youth. Having different funding streams and administrative requirements further impedes cross-system collaboration and the development of integrated treatment services.

To aid needed coordination between service systems, the severity of impairments related to each problem or diagnosis rather than diagnosis alone should be the basis of integrated treatment. Such an integrated model recommends moving toward greater integration as the severity of the co-occurring disorder(s) increases. A continuum of care can be based on the level of provider behavior (Hawkins, 2009). Levels along this continuum include (1) minimal coordination, (2) consultation: an informal exchange of clinical information and clinical recommendations often short of actual treatment, and (3) collaboration: a more structured arrangement involving regular, planned communication, often based on contractual agreements between systems or providers. Finally, and perhaps the most desirable level of care, is full integration. A fully integrated model refers to the development of a single treatment plan that addresses both mental health and SUDs concurrently by the same clinician(s) and at the same clinical venue.

Existing integrated practices consist of two general approaches. The first is treatment planning and care coordination, in which individual services, usually separate, are provided to best meet the needs of each adolescent and his or her family. The second approach includes evidence-based interventions that concurrently address psychiatric and substance abuse disorders.

The numerous needs of youth with comorbid disorders often extend beyond the treatment of SUDs and behavioral or emotional problems. They can include school and other environmental obstacles with multiple services targeted at the comorbid disorders. The use of intensive case management facilitates a coordinated treatment approach with or without integrated intervention programs. For adolescents with co-occurring disorders, this may include developing and monitoring a comprehensive service plan, providing support services to the client and his or her family, and crisis intervention and advocacy services as needed.

"Wraparound" is a model of care coordination for children and youth with mental health problems who are also involved with one or more other systems (e.g., child welfare, juvenile justice, special education). Wraparound requires a team-based planning process through which families, formal supports, and natural supports develop, monitor, and evaluate an individualized plan. While this can improve coordination of SUDs and psychiatric treatment, it does not necessitate integrated treatment.

APPROACHES TO THE TREATMENT OF COMORBID DISORDERS IN ADOLESCENTS

Treatment planning for adolescents with significant comorbidity involves a modest modification from that of SUDs alone. Similar to the primary elements of effective SUD treatment alone, the elements of dual-disorder treatment include:

1. Comprehensive assessment of behavioral, emotional, and substance use domains.
2. Engagement with adolescent and parents.

3. Maximized motivation to change.
4. Reduction of behavioral and/or emotional target behaviors and symptoms.
5. Development and maintenance of a prosocial and healthy lifestyle.
6. Relapse prevention.

Previous chapters in this book have discussed most of these elements in detail. Because multiple problems are often present in adolescents presenting for treatment, this approach and application of these elements is applicable and recommended for all teens.

Debate often arises as to which problem disorder should be treated first in adolescents with co-occurring disorders—substance use or other psychiatric disorder. The answer should be concurrent treatment, but there are no hard-and-fast rules. Given the availability of both SUD and psychiatric treatments in a specific locality, the priority target is usually determined by the severity of a particular problem and its effects on impairment, distress, and/or physical health. For example, suicidal behavior, particularly an attempt with medically severe sequelae, demands immediate attention before SUD interventions. Similarly, the presence of withdrawal symptoms from regular substance use with medical complications prompts a primary focus. Depending on the initial provider seeing the adolescent, clinician opinion or bias toward the importance of one problem over another may dictate which problem gets first attention.

The use of a paradigm in which one or the other problem—an SUD or a psychiatric disorder—is judged to be more important by virtue of the chronological order of onset is rarely helpful in my experience, and there is no research supporting its helpfulness. If neither the SUD nor the psychiatric disorder is more severe than the other, the best strategy is to give primary attention to the problem the adolescent considers most salient. Since many adolescents with co-occurring disorders do not recognize their substance use as a problem, integrated services may offer an opportunity to engage and motivate youth in treatment, ostensibly for the comorbid problem. Additional supportive services can then be offered.

> "It sounds like you are not really concerned about your marijuana use, but you *are* bothered by the depression and anxiety that you have been having for the past year or so? Maybe we can start by discussing ways to deal with the depression and anxiety."

The focus here is the adolescent's choice; the distress caused by internalizing disorders is seen as more important to the adolescent than the SUD. Because of typical problems with insight, primary attention to externalizing problems is less likely to come from the adolescent. However, an adolescent may see poor problem solving and poor anger control as issues to be addressed. These particular issues are common to both SUD and psychiatric disorders, and they are subsumed into most adolescent SUD CBT curricula.

"Given the kinds of trouble you have gotten into, it seems like your impulsivity—acting before thinking—gets you into most of these problems. Many kids who see me often report similar problems as well as difficulties making the right decisions or getting angry too easily. What about you?"

These major areas of intervention—SUD, internalizing symptoms, and/or externalizing behaviors—can be presented to the adolescent as a menu. When the comorbid psychiatric problem is chosen as the primary target of intervention, the astute clinician then incorporates attention to the SUD into the approach.

Recently, several attempts at integrated treatments for adolescents with SUDs and depression, PTSD, bipolar disorder, and suicidal behavior have provided models for both investigators and clinicians (Goldstein et al., 2014; Esposito-Smythers, Spirito, Kahler, Hunt, & Monti, 2011; Curry, Wells, Lochman, Craighead, & Nagy, 2003; Bukstein & Horner, 2010). Generally, these involve extending an existing evidenced-based treatment for one aspect of the comorbidity to another. For example, CBT for depression is expanded to include modules on substance use, and family therapy for SUDs is extended to include other deviant behaviors. Of course, existing evidence-based treatments, such as family therapy or CBT for problem solving, already target general factors that increase risk for multiple problems.

Among the issues faced in the development and delivery of these interventions as part of psychiatric treatment are choice of format—group, individual, or family—the use of urine drug screens, the level of confidentiality, minimal motivation, and selection of target-specific behaviors and cognitions. Adolescents with comorbid SUDs and psychopathology are among the most difficult youths to work with due to their combination of internalizing and externalizing symptoms and higher impairment; multiple risk factors across family, individual, peer, and community domains; and their poor insight and motivation. An attempt to combine these needs and targets under a single paradigm has simplified treatment, allowing focus on the following:

- Motivation.
- Behavioral and emotional management.
- Identification of triggers for substance use.

- Prosocial activities and peers.
- Psychoeducation.
- Pharmacotherapy.

Motivation

Many emotional and behavior problems can negatively affect motivation. For example, the neurovegetative symptoms such as angeria seen with depression, cognitive preoccupation, social isolation, and avoidance seen with depression, and or anxiety may retard treatment seeking and cooperation. For adolescent behavioral disorders such as ADHD and conduct disorder, the presence of such cognitive distortions as negative attributional bias and positive illusory bias on the one hand inhibits insight into personal control and responsibility for behavior, thus affecting motivation for change. On the other hand, the internal distress seen with mood and anxiety disorders may promote treatment seeking.

Using an MI approach, the clinician initially focuses on establishing empathy in engaging with the adolescent, promoting the consideration of behavioral and emotional problems and its relationship with substance use as a cause for concern and a target for change. In my experience, adolescents tend to be more interested in changing their mood states and general behavior and its consequences than in changing their substance use. Connecting the two problems—behavioral and emotional problems and substance use—often provides the path to change. For example, using MI, particularly OARS, to elicit current internalizing (mood and anxiety) or behavior problems and desire to change these, regardless of the adolescent's feelings or insight about his or her substance use, is a useful technique for dealing with adolescents with SUD–psychiatric comorbidity.

ADOLESCENT: I feel like crap most of the time. My friends tell me I am cranky—an asshole. I get angry pretty easily.

CLINICIAN: It sounds like you don't like the way that you feel!

ADOLESCENT: Hell no! I don't like this at all.

CLINICIAN: What affects the way you feel?

ADOLESCENT: School, sometimes my friends, and especially my parents.

CLINICIAN: What would happen if you were to feel differently, feel better?

ADOLESCENT: I think I would or might get along with folks better.

CLINICIAN: Any thoughts as to what you might do to feel better?

ADOLESCENT: I don't know—I guess go to therapy.

CLINICIAN: Well, one option is therapy. Is it OK if I tell you some options that other kids your age have found useful in getting their mood under control?

ADOLESCENT: OK, I guess.

CLINICIAN: Talk therapy—either by yourself or in a group of other kids with similar problems—is one way. Some kids find medication useful, and many do both.

ADOLESCENT: I can think about that, but I don't like telling others my business, and I know my cousin took medication and said that she did better.

CLINICIAN: OK, some kids say that changes in their lifestyle help.

ADOLESCENT: What do you mean?

CLINICIAN: Changing sleep habits, getting on a regular schedule. You had previously mentioned that you use marijuana several times a week. Does that affect your mood?

ADOLESCENT: It usually helps chill me out, but I sometimes can get very irritable the next day after using a lot, or some weeks it has gotten me very anxious. I think I had some panic attacks.

CLINICIAN: It sounds like marijuana use is sometimes good but often bad. What would you like to do about it?

ADOLESCENT: I don't know. I think I did feel better when I wasn't using last year when I couldn't use for a while. But what am I going to do for fun, do with my friends?

CLINICIAN: Friends and fun are very important to you, but you are still concerned about how you feel. Do you feel like you have any options?

ADOLESCENT: Well, not all my friends use, and I guess I could cut down my use?

Using MI to create discrepancy with the ways the adolescent feels—or behaves—and the way he or she wants to feel and behave is important in promoting motivation to change substance use. In the above example, the clinician utilizes selective, amplified, and double-sided reflections. The decisional balance exercise allows the clinician and adolescent to explore both the positives and negatives of the status quo—substance use versus change (not using).

CLINICIAN: So, one of the positives or advantages that you report from using is that it "chills" you, calms you down, so you don't feel so anxious in interacting with your friends or other random people that you meet. But one of the disadvantages is that you don't do very well with being with other people when you are not using or high. And one of the advantages of change is that you might be able to interact without using—because you can't be using or high *all* the time.

ADOLESCENT: Yeah, it works while I'm using but it's worse when I don't. Maybe I can't learn not to be anxious as long as I am using.

Behavioral and Emotional Management

Most of the evidence base in treating adolescents with internalizing disorders such as mood and anxiety is composed of adaptations of CBT. While the focus of CBT for depression and anxiety disorders is different from that of CBT for SUDs in adolescents, the formats are often similar enough for modules for internalizing problems to be subsumed into a single CBT curriculum. In fact, many of the current versions of CBT for adolescent SUD include modules on anger recognition and management and depression management due to the frequent occurrence of these problems in many adolescent SUD treatment populations. One session of CBT may not be enough to thoroughly cover each topic, and so the clinician needs to determine the intensity of attention to specific internalizing problems. Many of the adolescent depression CBT curricula have become modular, and modules can be selected as needed for the specific adolescent. For comorbid depression, the clinician might add CBT modules on suicidality, behavioral activation, and scheduling. Similarly, anxiety modules can also be added for social avoidance, exposure, and relaxation training on a case-by-case basis. These CBT modules can be tied to those modules dealing with substance use because they all help to decrease adverse internal states. This should increase adolescent interest in controlling substance use.

A variety of CBT strategies are used for both SUDs and internalizing problems; I attempt to tie the various modules together through identification of triggers and use of the problem-solving paradigm. For example, to treat comorbid conditions, clinicians can augment a specific CBT curriculum with several sessions focusing on how substance use contributes to anxiety and depression and vice versa through a functional analysis of substance use, identification of triggers for use, coping with cravings, refusal skills, and planning for emergencies and coping with relapse. Augmented sessions for comorbidity include evidence-based techniques such as exposure and relaxation training for anxiety disorders and CBT and/or DBT for depression. The emphasis depends on the severity of each comorbid problem, the focus of the clinician and/or treatment program (i.e., psychiatric vs. SUD treatment programs), and a collaborative decision by the adolescent and clinician.

> CLINICIAN: We have talked a bit about how depression and anxiety are triggers for your marijuana use.
>
> ADOLESCENT: Yes, I put them on my trigger list.
>
> CLINICIAN: What about triggers for your depression and anxiety? Let's start with anxiety. On days that you use, are there any special triggers for becoming anxious?
>
> ADOLESCENT: Well, before I use, I think about going out into public— being in school or hanging out, especially around a lot of people— that makes me anxious. So, I want to use just to feel calm.
>
> CLINICIAN: How well does it work? We know that anxiety is a trigger.
>
> ADOLESCENT: OK while I am high, but then I am even more anxious the next time—or when the high wears off. I don't think I can do it without being high.
>
> CLINICIAN: Maybe we need to look at alternative ways of controlling your anxiety so that you are calm—preferably without using.

For externalizing disorder comorbidities, attention to impulsivity, poor problem solving, and poor anger control are already covered in most versions of adolescent SUD CBT. Specific sessions on anger awareness and management and problem solving address common characteristics of adolescents with SUDs that likely reinforce substance use behavior. The clinician can look at a number of sources for details on additional modules (Curry et al., 2003; Esposito-Smythers, Spirito, Uth, & Lachance, 2006; Spirito, Esposito-Smythers, Wolff, & Uhl, 2011). A more or less complete list of potential CBT modules addressing comorbid psychiatric problems/disorders includes:

- Problem solving (see Chapter 6).
- Anger management.
- Mood management.
- Anxiety management.
- Dealing with nonsuicidal self-injurious behaviors (SIBs).
- Dealing with suicidal thoughts and behavior.
- Dealing with trauma.

Problem solving and anger management are so ubiquitous among adolescents with SUDs that a group format might be best. The other topics may be best delivered individually. Within an integrated framework, the clinician or program could intersperse individual sessions with group sessions using the same general format.

It's critically important for the clinician to bring substance use behaviors, triggers, and consequences into each of the comorbid psychiatric topics (e.g., depression, anxiety, ADHD) and constituent sessions whenever possible. For example, rather than substance use being the cause of all problems, substance use becomes a trigger or consequence and a problem to be solved on the way to management of mood, anxiety, and behavior. Let's examine session outlines for anger, depression, and anxiety. In the sample sessions in Tables 9.1, 9.2, and 9.3, the general format is the same as for the skills sessions in Chapter 6. It remains the same across sessions, with each session beginning with (1) a review of client status, which for the comorbid patient includes both (a) substance use and (b) depression and/or anxiety symptoms, general functioning, and well-being; and (2) use of skills discussed in previous session(s) and homework. I will focus on (3) the introduction of the new skill; (4) guidelines to use of each skill, role model, and role plays; (5) group exercises; and (6) suggested homework for the session. The clinician should integrate sessions from SUD cognitive-behavioral recovery skills (Chapter 6) with these anger, depression, and anxiety sessions. The order of these sessions is determined by the clinician's acumen. Considerations for ordering include adolescent priorities or preferences, severity of SUD versus psychiatric symptoms/ behaviors, and opportunity, that is, what seems most relevant or motivating depending on what is occurring in the adolescent's life such as starting a new school year, an interpersonal loss or social disappointment, or traumatic event. These modules should take at least two and perhaps more sessions, depending on how the adolescent assimilates and masters the material and demonstrates his or her ability to use these skills in practice and homework.

Integrated SUD Treatment and Anger Management

As is true of most of the skills sessions for adolescents and their parents, the introduction of each topic begins with psychoeducation or an explanation of the importance of each topic. For anger, the clinician first defines anger. In the development of anger control skills, awareness of anger is critical and includes a review of the triggers of anger, the manifestations or signs of anger, and the consequences of the anger—the ABC's of anger as a behavior. As much as possible, the clinician should prompt consideration of substance use in being a trigger, affecting the actual display of anger (e.g., the adolescent is more "out of control" if he or she is angry

TABLE 9.1. Integrated SUD Treatment and Anger Management Session

Session 1: Awareness of anger

- Introduction of new skill and rationale for use.
  - □ Anger as a normal emotion with the potential for harm.
  - □ Anger as a feeling (that we can handle through constructive communication) versus anger behavior with negative consequences (violence and harm to self or others).
  - □ Anger as a signal of a problem (situation).
  - □ Anger as a trigger—prelude to substance use, SIBs, or suicidal behavior.

- Skill-use guidelines.
  - □ Anger awareness.
    - Be aware of how you feel.
      Exercise: Anger as a trigger. The adolescent and clinician develop a list of common feelings, both positive and negative. Ask how these feelings affect the adolescent's thoughts and behavior (specifically, substance use or aggressive behavior).
    - Be aware of what is happening.
      —Adult demands, conflicts (with peers and/or adults).
      —Disappointment, frustration.
  - □ What can one do? Use of the problem-solving paradigm/steps regarding types of responses—aggressive, passive, and assertive.
  - □ Model example—demonstrate aggressive, passive, and assertive responses.
  - □ Role play—the adolescent shows examples of aggressive, passive, and assertive responses.
  - □ Homework and real-life practice exercises.
    - Feelings log—adolescent keeps track of episodes of angry feelings.

Session 2: Dealing with anger

- Introduction of new skill and rationale for use.
  - □ Anger management: the importance of dealing with anger.
  - □ How has anger gotten the adolescent in trouble? How has it bothered the adolescent?

- Skill-use guidelines.
  - □ Using self-talk to calm oneself down.
    - Think of phrases, words to calm oneself down.
    - Use problem-solving steps.
  - □ Relaxation training.

- Model example—demonstrate use of problem-solving steps.

- Role play—have the adolescent "think aloud" about using problem-solving steps.

- Homework (reminder) sheets and real-life practice exercises.
  - □ Track anger episodes and use of the techniques above.

TABLE 9.2. Integrated SUD Treatment and Depression Management (Two to Four Sessions)

- Introduction of new skill and rationale for use.
  - □ Automatic thoughts (cognitions) can lead to negative emotional states.
  - □ Adverse emotional states often trigger substance use.
  - □ Substance can produce both pleasant and adverse emotional states, but usually the latter over the long term.
  - □ Participation in pleasant and enjoyable activities (other than substance use) can improve mood.
- Skill-use guidelines—modeling and role playing.
  - □ Awareness: Pay attention to your mood.
  - □ Awareness: Pay attention to negative and self-defeating thoughts.
    - Symptoms of depression.
    - Negative cognitions (automatic negative thoughts).
      - —Overgeneralization.
      - —All-or-nothing thinking.
      - —Either–or thinking.
      - —Jumping to conclusions.
      - —Magnifying.
      - —Minimizing.
      - —Personalizing.
      - —Self-blame.
      - —Taking events out of context.
      - —Catastrophizing.
  - □ Answering negative thoughts.
    - Examining and challenging the evidence for a specific thought. For example:
      - —"Is there substantial evidence for my thought(s)?"
      - —"Is there evidence contrary to my thought(s)?"
      - —"What would someone else say about this?"
      - —"What is the worst-case scenario?"
      - —"Am I confusing a thought with fact?"
      - —"Will this matter in a week, a month, or a year?"
  - □ Increasing involvement in positive, pleasurable activities.
    - Daily activities—eating, sleeping.
    - Pleasurable activities—for example, exercise, video games, movies.
    - Mastery activities—for example, schoolwork, job, hobby, volunteer work.
  - □ Unpleasant activities—how to avoid in an appropriate manner.
- Group exercise: Think of something that makes you sad, identify automatic thoughts, and determine if they are valid.
- Homework and real-life practice exercises: Keep a feelings log, record feelings, precipitants, accompanying thoughts, and resulting behavior.

TABLE 9.3. Integrated SUD Treatment and Anxiety Management (Two to Four Sessions)

- Introduction of new skill and rationale for use.
  - Anxiety is a common trigger and consequence for substance use and relapse.
  - Like depression and other emotional states, anxiety is often caused by automatic negative cognitions.

- Skill-use guidelines—modeling and role playing.
  - Awareness of anxiety and fears.
    - Describe/identify anxiety feelings.
      —Relationship with substance use (as triggers and consequence).
    - Identify situations avoided due to anxiety.
  - Present material for cognitive restructuring: identifying and challenging negative cognitions.
    - Identify negative cognitions/self-talk related to anxiety.
    - Discuss support or lack of support for cognitions/self-talk.
      —Alternative explanations.
    - Behavioral experiments to test cognitive distortions (also involves exposure).
  - Relaxation training: progressive muscle relaxation or deep breathing.
  - Self-talk.
  - Create a fear or anxiety hierarchy.
    - Create a list of scary (anxiety-provoking) situations ranging from a little scary to unbearably scary.
  - Work through fear hierarchy—exposure with relaxation training.
    - Use anxious thoughts (in office) or actual exposure.
    - Stay in each scary situation until your fears subside.
    - Use relaxation training techniques and self-talk.

- Session exercises.
  - Identify and make a list of fears and accompanying negative thoughts.
  - Demonstrate and practice relaxation techniques.
  - Exposure in office (thinking about anxiety situations).

- Homework and real-life practice exercises.
  - Choose one or two items on the anxiety hierarchy and test exposure with relaxation.
  - Keep a feelings log; record feelings, precipitants, accompanying thoughts, and resulting behavior.

while using"), and as some of the consequences of an anger episode (e.g., "I want to control anger by using substances more"). The prevention of anger episodes, which are often accompanied by impulsivity and feeling "out of control," involves the early and immediate identification of triggers. Anger can be a trigger for substance use but also a consequence due to substance use; each possibility should be considered in sessions. The clinician assists the adolescent in making a comprehensive list of triggers for anger and reviews this list at every opportunity in order to allow the adolescent to develop the ability to abort anger episodes early or even before they occur. In the development of coping strategies as part of the problem-solving paradigm, possible responses to triggers are considered and more adaptive, prosocial responses are identified as preferred responses. With repeated examples and role plays, the adolescent develops an internal script in which he or she rapidly identifies triggers and almost automatically engages an optimal response.

> CLINICIAN: OK, you told me that you had an incident with your parents when you came home late.
>
> ADOLESCENT: Yeah, I missed curfew by a half hour, and I blew up when they grounded me for a week.
>
> CLINICIAN: Any other options for how you respond when the trigger of parental punishment occurs? We actually discussed this before, with the trigger being parent reaction to home rule violation. Do you remember possible responses to this trigger?
>
> ADOLESCENT: I could lose it and have a fit—I did that over the weekend. I could just accept it and move on. I could mention that I want to discuss changing the curfew rule—but in a calm way.
>
> CLINICIAN: I think we need to be more aware of the triggers that we identified and our responses that we previously discussed. Let's go over some role plays with other triggers that you identified and see if you remember your planned response—other than anger.

Integrated SUD Treatment and Depression Management

Table 9.2 presents an outline for depression management. Familiarity with CBT for depression is essential. The difference between CBT for depression with integrated CBT is the emphasis on substance use as potentially both a trigger for and a consequence of negative affective states. Similar to the approach to anger control, integrated CBT initially focuses on increasing adolescent awareness of negative mood states. Like CBT for depression, the clinician focuses on additional awareness and management of negative cognitions (e.g., overgeneralization or either–or thinking) that result from or contribute to negative mood states, which in turn result from or contribute to substance use. Similar to CBT for depression, the clinician assists the adolescent in examining and challenging the evidence for negative thoughts. Beyond the basic goal of identifying negative mood states as triggers for substance use, the clinician assists the adolescent in developing alternatives to substance use in response to the trigger of negative mood states. Behavioral activation or increasing participation in positive, pleasurable activities may serve to increase adolescent involvement in positive, prosocial activities and not deviant behaviors, including substance use.

Integrated SUD Treatment and Anxiety Management

In addition to the increasing awareness of anxiety and avoidant behaviors (e.g., skipping class due to social anxiety) as a trigger and consequences in relation to substance use, the clinician needs to both increase the adolescent's anxiety tolerance and also decrease anxiety upon exposure to the trigger. Like CBT for anxiety, the adolescent works through a fear or anxiety hierarchy, initially focusing on tolerating anxious thoughts, practice/role-play anxiety situations, and finally exposure to the real situation. Concurrently, the clinician teaches relaxation training in order for the adolescent to tolerate progressive exposure to his or her fear hierarchy.

Modifications of CBT for problems such as suicidal behavior, non-suicidal SIBs, and mood dysregulation include DBT (Miller, Rathus, & Linehan, 2007). In DBT, the clinician stance is one of not allowing substance use as it interferes with therapy. DBT is also skills oriented and includes behavioral analysis and problem solving. The four basic skills modules of DBT are mindfulness, interpersonal relations, emotion regulation, and distress tolerance. Finally, anxiety, emotional dysregulation, and a history of trauma are primary features of PTSD and are also a fairly common problem among adolescents with SUDs. Therapies such as trauma-focused CBT (Cohen, Mannarino, & Berliner, 2010) are also skills based, with component skills expanded to include stress inoculation through breathing and relaxation techniques, direct discussion of the traumatic experience, cognitive restructuring, and safety skills building. Seeking Safety is an integrated intervention for those with PTSD and SUDs with four content areas: cognitive, behavioral, interpersonal, and case management (Najavits et al., 2006).

As with depression and anxiety, the severity of PTSD, including the accompanying distress and psychosocial impairments, often necessitates adding SUD-related modules to the core therapy sessions. Again, the clinician needs to identify and emphasize that anxiety and mood symptoms can be triggers for substance use and relapse and that decreasing use or abstinence helps control anxiety and mood symptoms.

Identification of Triggers for Substance Use or Relapse to Use

Already a part of adolescent SUD CBT, the skill of identification of triggers for substance use or relapse to use can be modified slightly to emphasize recognizing internal states as triggers. Both acute and ongoing strategies can be developed for dealing with these triggers.

Prosocial Activities and Peers

Both in adolescent treatment groups and associated peer activities, adolescents with SUDs have an opportunity to test their distorted cognitions related to mood and anxiety symptoms. Adolescents also have the opportunity to test behavioral controls and social problem-solving skills in prosocial settings. Ask the adolescent to sample prosocial activities and then help evaluate his or her reactions. These samplings can be seen as tests for the adolescent. When successful, these activities and relationships can lead to increased involvement in prosocial activities with prosocial peers.

Psychoeducation

Providing adolescents and their parent(s) with information about comorbid disorders and their relationship with substance use and SUDs is important not only for informed consent but also for understanding how treatment addresses emotional and behavioral problems that the adolescent is more motivated to change. Many families want simple explanations as well as simple solutions. Because the relationship between substance use and mental health symptoms is complex and not fully understood, the clinician is advised not to provide a glib, simplistic explanation. A search for the underlying reason for the adolescent's substance use may be misplaced and perhaps overemphasizes substance use as self-medication. This can encourage a reliance on psychopharmacological treatments alone. That being said, it is important to acknowledge that an important interaction usually exists between psychiatric symptoms and substance use. The following points form a basis for an ongoing conversation about what the adolescent and his or her family believe the SUD–psychiatric disorder relationship is for them. Ultimately, their belief in an explanation may help or hinder motivation and compliance in a treatment plan.

What to tell adolescents and their families about comorbidity:

1. Adolescents with SUDs are more likely than those teens without SUDs to have psychiatric disorders such as depression, bipolar disorder, anxiety disorders, as well as behavior problems such as ADHD and conduct disorder.
2. The onset of SUDs can come before or after that of the psychiatric disorder. However, behavioral problems almost always precede the onset of SUDs.
3. There is often a reciprocal relationship in which substance use reinforces psychiatric symptoms, which, in turn, reinforces substance use.
4. Treating the first disorder (e.g., depression or ADHD) will prob-

ably not cure the second (SUD) without specific treatment for the second disorder.

I advise clinicians to complement structured or informal verbal psychoeducation with brochures from such organizations as the National Institutes of Health and the American Psychiatric Association (see the resources in the Appendix).

Psychoeducation should not be the sole basis for treatment. One drawback of psychoeducation is a tendency to label symptoms and behaviors. As I discussed previously, labeling may retard the motivation of adolescents or parents who do not wish to accept a particular label—hence, the potential value of an integrated approach, where labeling is much less important.

Pharmacotherapy

The use of medications in the treatment of adolescents with SUDs largely involves youth with comorbid psychiatric disorders. The decision to initiate medication should be based on a comprehensive psychiatric assessment, identifying specific targets that have an evidence-based treatment with medications. The use of psychotherapeutic and medication interventions for adolescents with SUD–psychiatric comorbidity may benefit the psychiatric and/or behavioral symptoms, but research does not support improvement in substance use behaviors without concurrent SUD treatment. With this consideration in mind, all adolescents, comorbid or not, should receive specific treatment targeted to their SUDs.

When considering medication, especially for comorbid psychiatric disorders, adolescents may receive mixed messages from family, friends, and others such as members of AA/NA. They may hear that medications are no different than any substance of abuse that modifies mood and perception or decreases anxiety. The idea of being drug free may extend to prescribed medications for specific psychiatric disorders rather than just abstinence from substances of abuse. Although this attitude has been diminishing over the past several decades, it is occasionally encountered by adolescents in treatment. The clinician must provide support for the teen and encourage compliance with the medication or a discussion with the prescribing physician as soon as possible. Even if the clinician is not the prescribing physician, checks on medication compliance by the clinician are useful.

While the potential use of illicit drugs or alcohol with pharmacotherapy demands medical oversight, the potential medical effects of previous substance use require a careful medical history and evaluation. Consistent with practice guidelines for psychopharmacotherapy, the prescriber should obtain informed consent from the adolescent and his or her parents to implement a medication trial using an adequate dose of the identified medication for an adequate duration of time. The prescriber also develops a plan to monitor the adolescent both short- and long-term.

Medications for ADHD

The mixed literature on the effectiveness of treating ADHD in patients with SUDs does not conclusively support specific drugs, time for initiation, or length of therapy, but open-label and randomized trials and clinical experience have provided some guidance. An important consideration for treatment is whether the patient has active, comorbid SUD, a history of SUD without active SUD, or neither an active SUD nor a history of SUD but past recreational use of drugs. A "history of SUD" is generally defined as a reasonable interval of remission of use or symptoms (at least 6–12 months).

- All adolescents with an SUD diagnosis should receive some form of SUD treatment.
- A subdiagnostic pattern of substance use, especially without impairment, suggests treatment consistent with those without an SUD.
- In adults with ADHD and active SUD symptoms, especially those with a stimulant or cocaine dependence and not receiving psychosocial SUD treatment, nonstimulants (atomoxetine, bupropion) are preferable to stimulants, given the absence of more substantial evidence of stimulant efficacy in this population.
- For those with active SUD with poor response to nonstimulants, especially if uncontrolled ADHD symptoms appear to contribute to relapse or instability of the SUD, the use of extended-release or longer-acting stimulants with lower abuse liability and diversion potential (see below) is a reasonable option but must be utilized under careful scrutiny and ongoing monitoring.
- Individuals whose SUD is stable or who have a past history of SUD may benefit from first-line stimulant treatment. Use of longer-acting or extended-release formulations of stimulants in this population would also be preferable.

SAFETY AND DIVERSION ISSUES FOR ADHD MEDICATIONS

The prevalence of stimulant abuse or dependence among adolescents with a history of ADHD and therapeutic stimulant use is very low. Although some commonly used pharmacological agents, such as stimulants, have inherent abuse potential (Bukstein, 2007), none of the controlled studies of medications for ADHD in individuals (adolescents and adults) with SUDs have identified significant safety or diversion issues. Despite few of the subjects being abstinent for substance use, there were a few serious adverse events. Nevertheless, stimulants may potentially be abused, and diversion has long been identified as an issue, particularly in younger students. The risk of diversion or misuse of a therapeutic agent by the adolescent, his or her peer group, or family members should prompt a thorough assessment of this risk. Risk factors include a history of abuse of the specific or other potentially abusable agents, a family or parental history of substance abuse, or antisocial behavior or antisocial personality disorder in the patient or family members. In the absence of clear evidence of ongoing misuse and reselling or high-risk situations, the potential for diversion should not be the sole reason for withholding stimulant medications. Rather, the clinician should always evaluate for these risk factors for diversion and set up a clear plan of control and administration of the stimulant (or other) medication. Clinicians should monitor prescriptions carefully, with high suspicion directed toward early requests for refills or lost prescriptions. The treating physician must require frequent follow-up for all adult ADHD-SUD patients; questionnaires, objective toxicology screens, and contingency plans are suggested. These patients may benefit from relapse prevention techniques that take their impulsivity into account. Other cognitive-behavioral approaches may also be useful.

Often, parental or adult supervision of medication administration can alleviate concerns about potential abuse. The clinician should also consider alternative agents to psychostimulants, such as atomoxetine or bupropion, which do not have abuse potential. The long-acting stimulant preparations (e.g., OROS methylphenidate, mixed amphetamine salts extended release, or lisdexamfetamine dimesylate) may offer less potential for abuse or diversion due to their form of administration, reduced level of reinforcement due to more gradual and longer time to maximum plasma concentration, and the ability to more easily monitor and supervise once-a-day dosing.

Medications for Mood and Anxiety Disorders

Many mood and anxiety symptoms in adolescents can be treated successfully with psychosocial methods such as CBT. Following current guidelines, mild to moderate depression without prior psychosocial treatment should be first treated with psychotherapy. Moderate to severe depression, particularly if complicated by psychosis or suicidal behavior, should prompt the use of antidepressants with therapy. A strong family history and past episodes of depression suggests a more aggressive medication approach. Among the existent antidepressants, none has a significant risk for abuse or diversion.

The approach for anxiety is similar. Exposure-based psychotherapies and CBT are good choices. Severe anxiety with substantial avoidance that interferes with social and school function may require medication. If pharmacotherapy is required, the use of selective serotonin reuptake inhibitors, tricyclic antidepressants, hydroxyzine, or buspirone is much preferred to the use of benzodiazepines.

What about Medications for Withdrawal?

Medications used to target alcohol-related cravings (e.g., naltrexone, acamprosate, and ondansetron) are increasingly used among adults and have been reported effective in adolescents. For the most part, their efficacy in adolescents has yet to be tested in controlled trials. The biggest exception is the use of buprenorphine for both withdrawal and maintenance therapy in opiate-dependent adolescents. Two controlled trials have established the value of buprenorphine in adolescents for acute and extended withdrawal, and a study for maintenance is expected in the future.

The use of buprenorphine for withdrawal in controlled settings (inpatient or under the supervision of a responsible adult) alleviates the need for multiple medications to control the various uncomfortable symptoms of opiate withdrawal. Its status as a "partial opiate agonist" means a lower risk of actual abuse and likely dependence, although diversion can be a problem. Unlike methadone, it can be given to adolescents, at least as young as 16 years old, by qualified physicians. For adolescents with opiate use disorder, serious consideration should be given to buprenorphine either as a withdrawal agent or as a maintenance medication. Although drug-free treatment might be a reasonable goal for an initial treatment attempt, the risk of recurrent relapse with opiates suggests buprenorphine maintenance after several adolescent treatment failures or relapses.

Naltrexone, acamprosate, ondansetron, and aversive agents such as disulfiram could be considered for use in treatment-resistant adolescents. Similarly, the use of medications to treat alcohol, benzodiazepine, or opiate withdrawal using medications, such as benzodiazepines (alcohol), clonidine, and buprenorphine (opiates), is not based on empirical research in adolescents but rather on research and experience with adults. Clinicians should use caution in considering pharmacological treatment for adolescents with comorbid SUDs and psychiatric disorders. The presence of SUDs or substance use may increase the potential for intentional or unintentional overdose with some psychotropic medications, especially in combination with some substances of abuse.

SUMMARY AND RECOMMENDATIONS

The "Practice Parameters for the Assessment and Treatment of Children and Adolescents with Substance Use Disorders" of the American Academy of Child and Adolescent Psychiatry (2005) set a minimum standard for SUD–psychiatric disorder comorbidity. Adolescents with SUDs should receive a thorough evaluation for comorbid psychiatric disorders, and, conversely, adolescents with psychiatric disorders should receive assessment for possible SUDs. Furthermore, comorbid disorders should be appropriately treated. As previously discussed, for severe presentation, this involves integration of treatment modalities rather than merely serial or concurrent treatment. However, acute stabilization of moderate to severe substance use problems may need to precede onset of attention to psychiatric comorbidity except for more severe presentations involving suicidal behavior and/or psychosis.

Critical elements of integrated treatment are motivation, family involvement, and the development of cognitive-behavioral skills. Emerging research and experience suggest that pharmacotherapy can be used safely and effectively in adolescents with SUDs, although not all studies have been consistently positive. However, pharmacotherapy has its limits, and all adolescents will need treatment that targets their substance use and related behaviors.

Epilogue

Throughout this book, I have provided clinical approaches to the assessment and treatment of adolescents with SUDs. Just as all adolescents are not the same, so, too, all adolescents with SUDs are not the same. They can be different in important ways that can greatly influence the course of SUDs and their response to treatment. To acquaint the reader with these differences, I included a discussion of the risk factors involved in the onset and maintenance of substance use in youth, as well as reviewed a variety of evidence-based intervention modalities. Rather than repeat detail and specific instructions, I have tried to focus on principles and outlines of approaches based on evidence-based practices as well as my own experience over the past 25 years. The reader potentially has access to detailed descriptions and manuals for many of the evidence-based practices. I encourage clinicians to examine these sources and, if interested, obtain training and supervision in order to become proficient in delivering these evidence-based practices.

While I have described components of an ideal, integrated intervention, the availability of specific treatment services for adolescents with SUD may be limited. The primary purpose of this book is to raise the familiarity and skill level of clinicians to be able to provide a satisfactory level of quality adolescent SUD treatment services. An individual clinician may be comfortable providing only some of these services, although to become as much of an expert as possible, I encourage further training and practice. At the very least, brief intervention provides a baseline level of intervention, adequate for some adolescents with mild-severity SUDs and serving as a segue to more intensive treatment. Modification of general family therapy and mental health interventions may also allow for an adequate dose.

PREVENTION

Prevention, especially tertiary prevention efforts, overlaps with treatment. Most prevention interventions are based on social learning models, including educational approaches, family-based interventions, and community-based projects (including school-based curricula and programs). Empirically based prevention efforts primarily involve strengthening resilience factors and reducing risk factors for the development of SUDs (National Institute on Drug Abuse, 2003; see Table E.1). Early intervention for psychopathology in youths at risk of SUDs (e.g., conduct disorder, ADHD, mood and anxiety disorders) is critical to prevent early-onset substance use and SUDs.

Primary and secondary prevention efforts using parent management training and family therapies are very similar to those for adolescent SUD with the goal of making changes in the environment that would reduce relevant risk factors for SUD, such as association with deviant peers and impaired family functioning.

When there is a heightened suspicion of substance use and associated problems, recommended psychoeducation can be provided in a group format with other parents, allowing for support and discussion. Support from professionals and parents will always be needed throughout the assessment and treatment process. Awareness of the nature of substance use problems in adolescents, including poor motivation, frequent relapses, and effects of comorbid psychopathology, may help to diminish parental distress. However, despite the information and skills to be conveyed to parents, professionals should always solicit and be cognizant of the parents' agenda. Parents may be more concerned about comorbid psychopathology or parent–adolescent conflict than concurrent substance use problems—or vice versa. Also, parents may have their own ideas for possible solutions but need permission to share them.

CONCLUSION

SUDs in adolescents is the result of an interaction of an array of risk factors ranging from genetically based traits to environmental influences. No two cases are exactly alike, and most have substantial differences, making

TABLE E.1. Principles for Effective Prevention Programs

Principle 1: Prevention programs should enhance protective factors and reverse or reduce risk factors.

Principle 2: Prevention programs should address all forms of drug abuse, alone or in combination, including the underage use of legal drugs (e.g., tobacco or alcohol); the use of illegal drugs (e.g., marijuana or heroin); and the inappropriate use of legally obtained substances (e.g., inhalants), prescription medications, or over-the-counter drugs.

Principle 3: Prevention programs should address the type of drug abuse problem in the local community, target modifiable risk factors, and strengthen identified protective factors.

Principle 4: Prevention programs should be tailored to address risks specific to population or audience characteristics, such as age, gender, and ethnicity, to improve program effectiveness.

Principle 5: Family-based prevention programs should enhance family bonding and relationships and include parenting skills; practice in developing, discussing, and enforcing family policies on substance abuse; and training in drug education and information.

Principle 6: Prevention programs can be designed to intervene as early as preschool to address risk factors for drug abuse, such as aggressive behavior, poor social skills, and academic difficulties.

Principle 7: Prevention programs for elementary school children should target improving academic and social-emotional learning to address risk factors for drug abuse, such as early aggression, academic failure, and school dropout. Education should focus on the following skills:

- Self-control.
- Emotional awareness.
- Communication.
- Social problem solving.
- Academic support, especially in reading.

Principle 8: Prevention programs for middle or junior high and high school students should increase academic and social competence with the following skills:

- Study habits and academic support.
- Communication.
- Peer relationships.
- Self-efficacy and assertiveness.
- Drug-resistance skills.
- Reinforcement of antidrug attitudes.
- Strengthening of personal commitments against drug abuse.

(continued)

234   *Epilogue*

TABLE E.1. *(continued)*

Principle 9: Prevention programs aimed at general populations at key transition points, such as the transition to middle school, can produce beneficial effects even among high-risk families and children. Such interventions do not single out risk populations and, therefore, reduce labeling and promote bonding to school and community.

Principle 10: Community prevention programs that combine two or more effective programs, such as family- and school-based programs, can be more effective than a single program.

Principle 11: Community prevention programs reaching populations in multiple settings—for example, schools, clubs, faith-based organizations, and the media—are most effective when they present consistent communitywide messages in each setting.

Principle 12: When communities adapt programs to match their needs, community norms, or differing cultural requirements, they should retain core elements of the original research-based intervention that include the following:

Structure (how the program is organized and constructed).

Content (what the information, skills, and strategies of the program are).

Delivery (how the program is adapted, implemented, and evaluated).

Principle 13: Prevention programs should be long-term, with repeated interventions (i.e., booster programs) to reinforce the original prevention goals. Research shows that the benefits from middle school prevention programs diminish without follow-up programs in high school.

Principle 14: Prevention programs should include teacher training on good classroom management practices, such as rewarding appropriate student behavior. Such techniques help to foster students' positive behavior, achievement, academic motivation, and school bonding.

Principle 15: Prevention programs are most effective when they employ interactive techniques, such as peer discussion groups and parent role playing, that allow for active involvement in learning about drug abuse and reinforcing skills.

Principle 16: Research-based prevention programs can be cost effective.

Source. Adapted from National Institute on Drug Abuse (2003).

a one-size-fits-all intervention approach often less than optimal. As we develop a more personalized approach to treatment of SUDs, attempting to match a variety of evidence-based interventions with salient targets, clinicians should feel increasingly confident that they can develop and maintain knowledge and skills to deliver some of these evidence-based treatments to adolescents and their families.

Resources

INTERNET RESOURCES

National Institute on Drug Abuse (NIDA)

www.drugabuse.gov

Resources for professionals, families, and adolescents about drugs of abuse, treatment, research, and science-based information about the health effects and consequences of drug abuse and addiction and resources for talking with kids about the impact of drug use on health.

National Institute on Alcohol Abuse and Alcoholism (NIAAA)

www.niaaa.nih.gov

Resources for professionals, families, and adolescents about alcohol, treatment, research, and science-based information about the health effects and consequences of alcohol and resources for talking with kids about the impact of alcohol use on health. Sections on underage drinking and "Alcohol Screening and Brief Intervention for Youth" (NIAAA, 2014).

Substance Abuse and Mental Health Services Administration (SAMHSA)

www.samhsa.gov

SAMHSA is the agency within the U.S. Department of Health and Human Services that leads public health efforts to advance the behavioral health of the nation. SAMHSA's mission is to reduce the impact of substance abuse and mental illness on America's communities. Sections of interest include the **Behavioral Health Treatment Services Locator:** Find alcohol and drug abuse treatment or mental health treatment facilities and programs around the country at *https://findtreatment.samhsa.gov*; and the **Evidence-Based Practices Web Guide:** features research findings and details about evidence-based practices used to prevent and treat mental and substance use disorders.

Drug Enforcement Agency (DEA)

www.dea.gov

Information about laws governing illicit drugs and fact sheets about specific drugs.

Centers for Disease Control and Prevention (CDC)

www.cdc.gov

The CDC website has reports about tobacco and smoking by youth as well as information about substance use in the context of other high-risk behaviors.

Partnership for Drug-Free Kids

www.drugfree.org

A nonprofit organization dedicated to reducing teen substance abuse and helping families impacted by addiction. The Partnership for Drug-Free Kids translates the science of teen drug use and addiction for families, providing parents with direct support to prevent and cope with teen drug and alcohol abuse. **Join Together** is a news aggregation service from the Partnership for Drug-Free Kids that provides daily or breaking news on the top substance abuse and addiction news that impacts work, life, and community. The news is pulled from a comprehensive search of the nation's leading broadcast, print and digital media

CASAColumbia

www.casacolumbia.org/addiction-research/reports/adolescent-substance-use

CASAColumbia informs Americans of the economic and social costs of addiction and risky substance use and its impact on their lives and assesses what works in prevention, treatment, and disease management.

Monitoring the Future (MTF)

www.monitoringthefuture.org

MTF is an ongoing study of the behaviors, attitudes, and values of American secondary school students, college students, and young adults. Each year, a total of approximately 50,000 8th-, 10th-, and 12th-grade students are surveyed. The website contains press releases, monographs, and other reports about this important annual survey of adolescent substance use.

The Lighthouse Institute

https://chestnut.org/li

Lighthouse Institute, a division of Chestnut Health Systems, Inc., was established in 1986. Its central mission is to help practitioners improve the quality of their services through research, training, and publishing. Featured programs include the Global Appraisal of Individual Needs (GAIN), a measure of substance use and related problems for evaluation and follow-up, and the Adolescent Community Reinforcement Approach (A-CRA), Community Reinforcement Approach (CRA), and Assertive Continuing Care (ACC).

TREATMENT MANUALS

Brent, D. A., Poling, K. D., & Goldstein, T. R. (2011). *Treating depressed and suicidal adolescents: A clinician's guide.* New York: Guilford Press.

Godley, S. H., Meyers, R. J., Smith, J. E., Karvinen, T., Titus, J. C., Godley, M. D., et al. (2001). *The adolescent community reinforcement approach for adolescent cannabis users* (Cannabis Youth Treatment Series, Vol. 4). Rockville, MD: U.S. Department of Health and Human Services, Substance Abuse and Mental Health Services Administration Center for Substance Abuse Treatment.

Liddle, H. A. (2001). *Multidimensional family therapy for adolescent cannabis users* (Cannabis Youth Treatment Series, Vol. 5). Rockville, MD: U.S. Department of Health and Human Services, Substance Abuse and Mental Health Services Administration Center for Substance Abuse Treatment.

Najavits, L. M. (2001). *Seeking safety: A treatment manual for PTSD and substance abuse.* New York: Guilford Press. Treatment website: *www.seekingsafety.org*

Sampl, S., & Kadden, R. (2001). *Motivational enhancement therapy and cognitive behavioral therapy for adolescent cannabis users: 5 sessions* (Cannabis Youth Treatment Series, Vol. 1). Rockville, MD: U.S. Department of Health and Human Services, Substance Abuse and Mental Health Services Administration Center for Substance Abuse Treatment.

Szapocznik, J., Hervis, O., & Schwartz, S. (2003). *Therapy manuals for drug addiction: Brief strategic family therapy for adolescent drug use.* (NIH Publication No. 03-4751). Washington DC: U.S. Department of Health and Human Services. Retrieved from *http://www.bsft.org/documents/BSFTNIDATherapyManual.pdf.*

Webb, C., Scudder, M., Kaminer, Y., & Kadden, R. (2001). *The motivational enhancement therapy and cognitive behavioral therapy supplement: 7 sessions of cognitive behavioral therapy for adolescent cannabis users* (Cannabis Youth Treatment Series, Vol. 2). Rockville, MD: U.S. Department of Health and Human Services, Substance Abuse and Mental Health Services Administration Center for Substance Abuse Treatment.

References

Alexander, J. F., & Parsons. B. V. (1982). *Functional family therapy: Principles and procedures.* Carmel, CA: Brooks/Cole.

Alexander, J. F., Waldon, H. B., Newberry, A. M., & Liddle, N. (1990). The functional family therapy model. In A. S. Friedman & S. Granick (Eds.), *Family therapy for adolescent drug abuse* (pp. 183–200). Lexington, MA: Lexington Books.

American Academy of Child and Adolescent Psychiatry. (2005). Practice parameters for the assessment and treatment of children and adolescents with substance use disorders. *Journal of the American Academy of Child and Adolescent Psychiatry, 44,* 609–621.

American Academy of Pediatrics (AAP). (2011). Substance use screening, brief intervention, and referral to treatment for pediatricians. *Pediatrics, 128,* e1330.

American Psychiatric Association. (2000). *Diagnostic and statistical manual of mental disorders* (4th ed., text rev.). Washington, DC: Author.

American Psychiatric Association. (2013). *Diagnostic and statistical manual of mental disorders* (5th ed.). Arlington, VA: Author.

American Society of Addiction Medicine. (2013). *The ASAM criteria: Treatment criteria for addictive, substance-related, and co-occurring conditions* (3rd ed.). Chevy Chase, MD: Author.

Armbruster, P., & Kazdin, A. (1994). Attrition in child psychotherapy. In T. H. Ollendick & R. J. Prinz (Eds.), *Advances in clinical child psychology* (Vol. 16, pp. 81–108). New York: Plenum Press.

Armstrong, T. D., & Costello, E. J. (2002). Community studies of adolescent substance use, abuse, or dependence and psychiatric comorbidity. *Journal of Consulting and Clinical Psychology, 70,* 1224–1239.

Arrazola, R. A., Singh, T., Corey, C. G., Husten, C. G., Neff, L. J., Apelberg, B. J., et al. (2015). Tobacco use among middle and high school students—United States, 2011–2014. *Morbidity and Mortality Weekly Report, 64*(14), 381–385.

Azrin, N. H., Donohue, B., Teichner, G. A., Crum, T., Howell, J., & DeCato, L. A. (2001). A controlled evaluation and description of individual-cognitive problem solving and family-behavior therapies in dually-diagnosed conduct-disordered and substance-dependent youth. *Journal of Child and Adolescent Substance Abuse, 11*, 1–43.

Barnett, E., Sussman, S., Smith, C., Rohrbach, L. A., & Spruijt-Metz, D. (2012). Motivational interviewing for adolescent substance use: A review of the literature. *Addictive Behaviors, 37*(12), 1325–1334.

Batalla, A., Bhattacharyya, S., Yücel, M., Fusar-Poli, P., Crippa, J. A., Nogué, S., et al. (2013). Structural and functional imaging studies in chronic cannabis users: A systematic review of adolescent and adult findings. *PLOS ONE, 8*, e55821.

Becker, S. J., & Curry, J. F. (2008). Outpatient interventions for adolescent substance abuse: A quality of evidence review. *Journal of Consulting and Clinical Psychology, 76*, 531–544.

Biederman, J., Wilens, T., Mick, E., Milberger, S., Spencer, T. J., & Faraone, S. V. (1995). Psychoactive substance use disorders in adults with attention deficit hyperactivity disorder (ADHD): Effects of ADHD and psychiatric comorbidity. *American Journal of Psychiatry, 152*(11), 1652–1658.

Bien, T. H., Miller, W. R., & Tonigan, J. S. (1993). Brief interventions for alcohol problems: A review. *Addiction, 88*, 305–325.

Brent, D. A., Poling, K. D., & Goldstein, T. R. (2011). *Treating depressed and suicidal adolescents: A clinician's guide.* New York: Guilford Press.

Brown, S. A. (2001). Facilitating change for adolescent alcohol problems: A multiple options approach. In E. F. Wagner & H. B. Waldron (Eds.), *Innovations in adolescent substance abuse interventions* (pp 169–187). Amsterdam: Pergamon/Elsevier Science.

Brown, S. A., D'Amico, E. J., McCarthy, D. M., & Tapert, S. F. (2001). Four-year outcomes from adolescent alcohol and drug treatment. *Journal of Studies on Alcohol, 62*(Suppl.), 381–388.

Brown, S. A., Gleghorn, A., Schuckit, M. A., Myers, M. G., & Mott, M. A. (1996). Conduct disorder among adolescent alcohol and drug abusers. *Journal of Studies on Alcohol, 57*, 314–324.

Brown, S. A., McGue, M., Maggs, J., Schulenberg, J., Hingson, R., Swartzwelder, S., et al. (2008). A developmental perspective on alcohol and youths 16 to 20 years of age. *Pediatrics, 121*, S290–S310.

Brown, S. A., Mott, M. A., & Myers, M. G. (1990). Adolescent alcohol and drug treatment outcome. In R. R. Watson (Ed.), *Drug and alcohol abuse prevention* (pp. 373–403). Totowa, NJ: Humana Press.

Brown, S. A., Myers, M. G., Mott, M. A., & Vik, P. W. (1994). Correlates of success following treatment for adolescent substance abuse. *Applied and Preventive Psychology, 3*, 61–73.

Brown, S. A., Tapert, S. F., Granholm, E., & Delis, D. C. (2000). Neurocognitive functioning of adolescents: Effects of protracted alcohol use. *Alcoholism: Clinical and Experimental Research, 24,* 164–171.

Bukstein, O. G. (1994). Substance abuse. In M. Hersen, R. T. Ammerman, & L. A. Sisson (Eds.), *Handbook of aggressive and destructive behavior in psychiatric patients* (pp. 445–468). New York: Plenum Press.

Bukstein, O. G. (1995). *Adolescent substance abuse: Assessment, treatment and prevention perspectives.* New York: Wiley.

Bukstein, O. G. (1996). Agression, violence and adolescent substance abuse. *Child and Adolescent Psychiatric Clinics of North America, 5,* 93–109.

Bukstein, O. G. (2007). Therapeutic challenges of attention-deficit hyperactivity disorder with substance use disorders. *Expert Review of Neurotherapeutics, 6,* 541–549.

Bukstein, O. G. (2008). Substance use disorders in adolescents with attention-deficit/hyperactivity disorder. *Adolescent Medicine, 19,* 242–253.

Bukstein, O. G. (2009). Adolescent substance Abuse. In B. J. Sadock, V. A. Sadock, & P. Ruiz (Eds.), *Comprehensive textbook of psychiatry* (9th ed., Vol. 2, pp. 3818–3833). Philadelphia: Wolters Kluwer/Lippincott Williams & Wilkins.

Bukstein, O. G. (2016). Conduct disorder and delinquency and substance use Disorders. In Y. Kaminer (Ed.), *Youth substance abuse and co-occurring disorders* (pp. 81–102). Arlington, VA: American Psychiatric Publishing.

Bukstein, O. G., Brent, D. A., & Kaminer, Y. (1989). Comorbidity of substance abuse and other psychiatric disorders in adolescents. *American Journal of Psychiatry, 146,* 1131–1141.

Bukstein, O. G., Brent, D. A., Perper, J. A., Moritz, G., Baugher, M., Schweers, J., et al. (1993). Risk factors for completed suicide among adolescents with a lifetime history of substance abuse: A case-control study. *Acta Psychiatrica Scandinavica, 88,* 403–408.

Bukstein, O. G., & Deas, D. (2009). Substance abuse and addictions. In M. K. Dulcan (Ed.), *Dulcan's textbook of child and adolescent psychiatry* (pp. 241–260). Washington, DC: American Psychiatric Press.

Bukstein, O. G., Glancy, L. J., & Kaminer, Y. (1992). Patterns of affective comorbidity in a clinical population of dually diagnosed adolescent substance abusers. *Journal of the American Academy of Child and Adolescent Psychiatry, 31*(6), 1041–1045.

Bukstein, O. G., & Horner, M. S. (2010). Management of the adolescent with substance use disorders and comorbid psychopathology. *Child and Adolescent Psychiatric Clinics of North America, 19*(3), 609–623.

Bukstein, O. G., & Tarter, R. (2005). Substance use disorders. In C. E. Coffey & R. A. Brumback (Eds.), *Pediatric neuropsychiatry* (pp. 321–341). Philadelphia: Lippincott Williams & Williams.

Carey, K. B., Scott-Sheldon, L. A., Carey, M. P., & DeMartini, D. S. (2007). Individual-level interventions to reduce college student drinking: A meta-analytic review. *Addictive Behaviors, 32,* 2469–2494.

Carney, T., & Myers, B. (2012). Effectiveness of early interventions for substance using adolescents: Findings from a systematic review and meta-analysis. *Sub-*

stance Abuse Treatment, Prevention, and Policy, 7, 25. Retrieved January 5, 2018 from *www.substanceabusepolicy.com/content/7/1/25.*

Carney, T., Myers, B. J., Louw, J., & Okwundu, C. I. (2014). Brief school-based interventions and behavioural outcomes for substance-using adolescents. *Cochrane Database of Systematic Reviews, 4*, 2.

Casey, B. J., & Jones, R. M. (2010). Neurobiology of the adolescent brain and behavior: Implications for substance use disorders. *Journal of the American Academy of Child and Adolescent Psychiatry, 49*(12), 1189–1201.

Center for Substance Abuse Treatment. (1999a). *Brief interventions and brief therapies for substance abuse* (Treatment Improvement Protocol 34, Report No. [SMA] 99-3353). Rockville, MD: U.S. Substance Abuse and Mental Health Services Administration.

Center for Substance Abuse Treatment. (1999b). *Treatment for stimulant use disorders* (Treatment Improvement Protocol 33, DHHS Publication No. [SMA] 09-4209). Rockville, MD: U.S. Substance Abuse and Mental Health Services Administration.

Chaffin, M., Silovsky, J., Funderburk, B., Valle, L. A., Brestan, E. V., Balachova, T., et al. (2004). Parent–child interaction therapy with physically abusive parents: Efficacy for reducing future abuse reports. *Journal of Consulting and Clinical Psychology, 72*, 491–499.

Chamberlain P., & Reid, J. B. (1998). Comparison of two community alternatives to incarceration for chronic juvenile offenders. *Journal of Consulting and Clinical Psychology, 66*(4), 624–633.

Chambless, D. L., & Hollon, S. (1998). Defining empirically supported therapies. *Journal of Consulting and Clinical Psychology, 66*, 7–18.

Chan, Y. F., Dennis, M. L., & Funk, R. R. (2008). Prevalence and comorbidity of major internalizing and externalizing problems among adolescents and adults presenting to substance abuse treatment. *Journal of Substance Abuse Treatment, 34*(1), 14–24.

Charach, A., Yeung, E., Climans, T., & Lillie, E. (2011). Childhood attention-deficit/hyperactivity disorder and future substance use disorders: Comparative meta-analyses. *Journal of the American Academy of Child and Adolescent Psychiatry, 50*, 9–21.

Chen, C., Wagner, F., & Anthony, J. (2002). Marijuana use and the risk of major depressive episode: Epidemiological evidence from the United States National Comorbidity Survey. *Social Psychiatry and Psychiatric Epidemiology, 37*, 199–206.

Chung, T. (2008). Adolescent substance use, abuse, and dependence: Prevalence, course, and outcomes. In Y. Kaminer & O. G. Bukstein (Eds.), *Adolescent substance abuse: Psychiatric comorbidity and high-risk behavior* (pp. 29–52). New York: Routledge/Taylor & Francis.

Chung, T., Maisto, S. A., Cornelius, J. R., & Martin, C. S. (2004). Adolescents' alcohol and drug use trajectories in the year following treatment. *Journal of Studies on Alcohol, 65*(1), 105–114.

Chung, T., & Martin, C. S. (2001). Classification and course of alcohol problems among adolescents in addictions treatment programs. *Alcoholism: Clinical and Experimental Research, 25*, 1734–1742.

Chung, T., & Martin, C. S. (2005). Classification and short-term course of DSM-IV cannabis, hallucinogen, cocaine, and opioid disorders in treated adolescents. *Journal of Consulting and Clinical Psychology, 73*(6), 995–1004.

Chung, T., & Martin, C. S. (2011). Adolescent substance use and substance use disorders: Prevalence and clinical course. In Y. Kaminer & K. C. Winters (Eds.), *Clinical manual of adolescent substance abuse treatment* (pp. 1–23). Arlington, VA: American Psychiatric Publishing.

Chung, T., Martin, C. S., Grella, C. E., Winters, K. C., Abrantes, A. M., & Brown, S. A. (2003). Course of alcohol problems in treated adolescents. *Alcoholism: Clinical and Experimental Research, 27*(2), 253–261.

Clark, D. B., Martin, C. S., Chung, T., Gordon, A. J., Fiorentino, L., Tootell, M., et al. (2016). Screening for underage drinking and DSM-5 alcohol use disorder in rural primary care practice. *Journal of Pediatrics, 173*, 214–220.

Clark, D. B., Pollock, N., Bukstein, O. G., Mezzich, A., Bromberger, J. T., & Donovan, J. E. (1997). Gender and comorbid psychopathology in adolescents with alcohol dependence. *Journal of the American Academy of Child and Adolescent Psychiatry, 36*, 1195–1203.

Cleveland, M. J., Feinberg, M. E., Bontempo, D. E., & Greenberg, M. T. (2008). The role of risk and protective factors in substance use across adolescence. *Journal of Adolescent Health, 43*, 157–164.

Cohen, J. A., Mannarino, A. P., & Berliner, L. (2010). Trauma-focused CBT for children with co-occurring trauma and behavioral problems. *Child Abuse and Neglect, 34*, 215–224.

Collier, C., Hilliker, R., & Onwuegbuzie, A. (2014). Alternative peer group: A model for youth recovery. *Journal of Groups in Addiction and Recovery, 9*, 40–53.

Cornelius, J. R., Maisto, S. A., Martin, C. S., Bukstein, O. G., Salloum, M., Daley, D. C., et al. (2004). Major depression associated with earlier alcohol relapse in treated teens with AUD. *Addictive Behaviors, 29*, 1035–1038.

Costa Dias, T. G., Wilson, V. B., Bathula, D. R., Iyer, S. P., Mills, K. L., Thurlow, B. L., et al. (2013). Reward circuit connectivity relates to delay discounting in children with attention-deficit/hyperactivity disorder. *European Neuropsychopharmacology, 23*(1), 33–45.

Cunningham, P. B., & Henggeler, S. W. (1999) Engaging multi-problem families in treatment: Lessons learned throughout the development of multisystemic therapy. *Family Process, 38*, 265–286.

Cunningham, R. M., Walton, M. A., Goldstein, A., Chermack, S. T., Shope, J. T., Bingham, C. R., et al. (2009). Three-month follow-up of brief computerized and therapist interventions for alcohol and violence among teens. *Academic Emergency Medicine, 16*, 1193–1207.

Curry, J. F., Wells, K. W., Lochman, J. E., Craighead, W. E., & Nagy, P. D. (2003). Cognitive behavioral intervention for depressed, substance abusing adolescents: Development and pilot testing. *Journal of the American Academy of Child and Adolescent Psychiatry, 42*, 656–665.

Dahl, R. E., & Spear, L. P. (Eds.). (2004). *Annals of the New York Academy of Sciences: Vol. 1021. Adolescent brain development: Vulnerabilities and opportunities.* New York: New York Academy of Sciences.

Dakof, G. A. (2000). Understanding gender differences in adolescent drug abuse: Issues of comorbidity and family functioning. *Journal of Psychoactive Drugs, 32*, 25–32.

D'Amico, E. J., Ellickson, P. L., Wagner, E. F., Turrisi, R., Fromme, K., Ghosh-Dastidar, B., et al. (2005). Developmental considerations for substance use interventions from middle school through college. *Alcoholism: Clinical and Experimental Research, 29*(3), 474–483.

Degenhardt, L., Coffey, C., Romaniuk, H., Swift, W., Carlin, J. B., Hall, W. D., et al. (2013). The persistence of the association between adolescent cannabis use and common mental disorders into young adulthood. *Addiction, 108*, 124–133.

Demos, J., & Demos, V. (2009). Adolescence in historical perspective. *Journal of Marriage and Family, 31*(4), 632–638.

Dennis, M. (1999). *Global appraisal of individual needs (GAIN): Administration guide for the GAIN and related measures.* Bloomington, IL: Chestnut Health Systems.

Dennis, M. L., Godley, S. H., Diamond, G., Tims, F. M., Babar, T., Donaldson, J., et al. (2004). The Cannabis Youth Treatment (CYT) Study: Main findings from two randomized trials. *Journal of Substance Abuse Treatment, 27*, 197–213.

DePanfilis, D. (2000). How do I develop a helping alliance with the family? In H. Dubowitz & D. DePanfilis (Eds.), *Handbook for child protection practice* (pp. 34–38). Newberry Park, CA: SAGE.

Diamond, G., Godley, S. H., Liddle, H. A., Sampl, S., Webb, C., Tims, F. M., et al. (2002). Five outpatient treatment models for adolescent marijuana use: A description of the Cannabis Youth Treatment Interventions. *Addiction, 97*(Suppl. 1), 70–83.

Donohue, B., & Azrin, N. H. (2011). *Family behavior therapy: A step-by-step approach to adolescent substance abuse.* Hoboken, NJ: Wiley.

Donohue, B., Azrin, N., Lawson, H., Friedlander, J., Teicher, G., & Rindsberg, J. (1998). Improving initial session attendance of substance abusing and conduct disordered adolescents: A controlled study. *Journal of Child and Adolescent Substance Abuse, 8*, 1–13.

Doran, N., Luczak, S. E., Bekman, N., Koutsenek, I., & Brown, S. A. (2012). Adolescent substance use and aggression: A review. *Criminal Justice and Behavior, 39*, 748–769.

Dutra, L. M., & Glantz, S. A. (2014). Electronic cigarettes and conventional cigarette use among US adolescents: A cross-sectional study. *Journal of the American Medical Association Pediatrics, 168*(7), 610–617.

Ercan, E. S., Coskunol, H., Varan, A., & Toksoz, K. (2003). Childhood attention deficit/hyperactivity disorder and alcohol dependence: A 1-year follow-up. *Alcohol, 38*, 352–356.

Erickson, S. J., Gerstle, M., & Feldstein, S. W. (2005). Brief interventions and motivational interviewing with children, adolescents, and their parents in pediatric health care settings: A review. *Archives of Pediatric Adolescent Medicine, 159*, 1173–1180.

Esposito-Smythers, C., Spirito, A., Kahler, C. W., Hunt, J., & Monti, P. (2011). Treatment of co-occurring substance abuse and suicidality among adolescents: A randomized trial. *Journal of Consulting and Clinical Psychology, 79,* 728–739.

Esposito-Smythers, C., Spirito, A., Uth, R., & Lachance, H. (2006). Cognitive behavioral treatment for suicidal alcohol abusing adolescents: Development and pilot testing. *American Journal on Addictions, 15*(Suppl.), 126–130.

Finch, A. J., Tanner-Smith, E., Hennessy, E., & Moberg, D. P. (2018). Recovery high schools: Effect of schools supporting recovery from substance use disorders. *American Journal of Drug and Alcohol Abuse, 44,* 175–184.

Flory, K., Milich, R., Lynam, D. R., Leukefeld, C., & Clayton, R. (2003). Relation between childhood disruptive behavior disorders and substance use and dependence symptoms in young adulthood: Individuals with symptoms of attention-deficit/hyperactivity disorder and conduct disorder are uniquely at risk. *Psychology of Addictive Behaviors, 17*(2), 151–158.

French, M. T., Zavala, S. K., McCollister, K. E., Waldron, H. B., Turner, C. W., & Ozechowski, T. J. (2008). Cost-effectiveness analysis (CEA) of four interventions for adolescents with a substance use disorder. *Journal of Substance Abuse Treatment, 34,* 272–281.

Godley, M. D., Godley, S. H., Dennis, M. L., Funk. R., & Passetti, L. (2002). Preliminary outcomes from the assertive continuing care experiment for adolescents discharged from residential treatment. *Journal of Substance Abuse Treatment, 23,* 21–32.

Godley, M. D., Godley, S. H., Dennis, M. L., Funk, R. R., & Passetti, L. L. (2007). The effect of assertive continuing care on continuing care linkage, adherence and abstinence following residential treatment for adolescents with substance use disorders. *Addiction, 102*(1), 81–93.

Godley, S. H., Garner, B. R., Passetti, L. L., & Funk, R. R. (2010). Adolescent outpatient treatment and continuing care: Main findings from a randomized clinical trial. *Drug and Alcohol Dependence, 110,* 44–54.

Godley, S. H., Meyers, R. J., Smith, J. E., Karvinen, T., Titus, J. C., Godley, M. D., et al. (2001). *The adolescent community reinforcement approach for adolescent cannabis users* (Cannabis Youth Treatment Series, Vol. 4). Rockville, MD: U.S. Department of Health and Human Services, Substance Abuse and Mental Health Services Administration Center for Substance Abuse Treatment.

Gogtay, N., Giedd, J. N., Lusk, L., Havashi, K. M., Greenstein, D., Vaituzis, A. C., et al. (2004). Dynamic mapping of human cortical development during childhood through early adulthood. *Proceedings of the National Academy of Sciences of the USA, 101*(21), 8174–8179.

Goldstein, A. P., Sprafkin, R. P., Gershaw, N. J., & Klein, P. (1980). *Skill-streaming the adolescent: A structured learning approach to teaching prosocial skills.* Champaign, IL: Research Press.

Goldstein, B. I., Goldstein, T. R., Collinger, K. A., Axelson, D. A., Bukstein, O. G., Birmaher, B., et al., (2014). Treatment development and feasibility study of family-focused treatment for adolescents with bipolar disorder and comorbid substance use disorders. *Journal of Psychiatric Practice, 20*(3), 237–248.

Goldston, D. B., Daniel, S. S., Mathias, C. W., & Dougherty, D. M. (2008). Suicidal and nonsuicidal self-harm behaviors in adolescent substance use disorders. In Y. Kaminer & O. G. Bukstein (Eds.), *Adolescent substance abuse: Psychiat-*

ric comorbidity and high-risk behaviors (pp. 323–354). New York: Routledge/ Taylor & Francis.

Grant, B. F., & Dawson D. A. (1998). Age of onset of drug use and its association with DSM-IV drug abuse and dependence: Results from the National Longitudinal Alcohol Epidemiologic Survey. *Journal of Substance Abuse, 10,* 163–173.

Gray, K. M., Carpenter, M. J., Baker, N. L., DeSantis, S. M., Kryway, E., Hartwell, K. J., et al. (2012a). Double-blind randomized controlled trial of N-acetylcysteine in cannabis-dependent adolescents. *American Journal of Psychiatry, 169,* 805–812.

Gray, K. M., Carpenter, M. J., Baker, N. L., Hartwell, K. J., Lewis, A. L., Hiott, D. W., et al. (2011). Bupropion SR and contingency management for adolescent smoking cessation. *Journal of Substance Abuse Treatment, 40,* 77–86.

Gray, K. M., Carpenter, M. J., Lewis, A. L., Klintworth, E. M., & Upadhyaya, H. P. (2012b). Varenicline versus Bupropion XL for smoking cessation in older adolescents: A randomized, double-blind pilot trial. *Nicotine and Tobacco Research, 14,* 234–239.

Grella, C., Hser, Y. I., Joshi, V., & Rounds-Bryant, J. (2001). Drug treatment outcomes for adolescents with comorbid mental and substance use disorders. *Journal of Nervous and Mental Diseases, 189,* 384–392.

Grenard, J. L., Ames, S. L., Pentz, M. A., & Sussman, S. (2006). Motivational interviewing with adolescents and young adults for drug related problems. *International Journal of Adolescent Medical Health, 18,* 53–67.

Gross, J., & McCaul, M. E. (1990–1991). A comparison of drug use and adjustment in urban adolescent children of substance abusers. *International Journal of the Addictions, 25,* 495–511.

Gustavson, D. E., Stallings, M. C., Corley, R. P., Miyake, A., Hewitt, J. K., & Friedman, N. P. (2017). Executive functions and substance use: Relations in late adolescence and early adulthood. *Journal of Abnormal Psychology, 126,* 257–270.

Hall, W., & Weier, M. (2017). Has marijuana legalization increased marijuana use among U.S. youth? *Journal of the American Medical Association Pediatrics, 171,* 116–118.

Hamilton, N., Brantley, L., Tims, F., Angelovich, N., & McDougall, B. (2001). *Family support network for adolescent cannabis users* (Cannabis Youth Treatment Series, Vol. 3). Rockville, MD: Center for Substance Abuse Treatment, Substance Abuse and Mental Health Services Administration.

Harrell, A. V., &, Wirtz, P. W. (1989). Screening for adolescent problem drinking: Validation of a multidimensional instrument for case identification. *Psychological Assessment: A Journal of Consulting and Clinical Psychology, 1,* 61–63.

Hawkins, E. (2009). A tale of two systems: Co-occurring mental health and substance abuse disorders treatment for adolescents. *Annual Review of Psychology, 60,* 197–227.

Hendriks, V., van der Schee, E., & Blanken, P. (2012). Matching adolescents with a cannabis use disorder to multidimensional family therapy or cognitive behavioral therapy: Treatment effects moderators in a randomized controlled trial. *Drug and Alcohol Dependence, 125,* 119–126.

Henggeler, S. W., Borduin, C. M., Melton, G. B., Mann, B. J., et al. (1991). Effects of multisystemic therapy on drug use and abuse in serious juvenile offenders: A progress report from two outcome studies. *Family Dynamics Addiction Quarterly, 1,* 40–51.

Henggeler, S. W., Cunningham, P. B., & Rowland, M. D. (2011). *Contingency management for adolescent substance abuse: A practitioner's guide.* New York: Guilford Press.

Henggeler, S. W., Halliday-Boykins, C. A., Cunningham, P. B., Randall, J., Shapiro, S. B., & Chapman, J. E. (2006). Juvenile drug court: Enhancing outcomes by integrating evidence-based treatments. *Journal of Consulting and Clinical Psychology, 74*(1), 42–54.

Henggeler, S. W., Pickrel, S. G., & Brondino, M. J. (1999). Multi-systemic treatment of substance abusing and dependent delinquents: Outcomes, treatment fidelity, and transportability. *Mental Health Services Research, 1,* 171–184.

Hibell, B., Guttormsson, U., Ahlström, S., Balakireva, O., Bjarnason, T., Kokkevi, A., & Kraus, L. (2009). *The 2007 ESPAD report: Substance use among students in 35 European countries.* Stockholm: Swedish Council for Information on Alcohol and Other Drugs.

Hogue, A., Henderson, C. E., Ozechowski, T. J., & Robbins, M. S. (2014). Evidence base on outpatient behavioral treatments for adolescent substance use: Updates and recommendations 2007–2013. *Journal of Clinical Child and Adolescent Psychology, 43,* 695–720.

Hser, Y. I., Grella, C. E., Hubbard, R. L., Hsieh, S. C., Fletcher, B. W., Brown, B. S., & Anglin, M. D. (2001). An evaluation of drug treatments for adolescents in four U.S. cities. *Archives of General Psychiatry, 58,* 689–695.

Hsieh, S., Hoffmann, N. G., & Hollister, C. D. (1998). The relationship between pre-, during-, post-treatment factors, and adolescent substance abuse behaviors. *Addictive Behaviors, 23,* 477–488.

Huizinga, D., Menard, S., & Elliott, D. S. (1989). Delinquency and drug use: Temporal and developmental patterns. *Justice Quarterly, 6,* 419–455.

Ives, M. L., Chan, Y.-F., Modisette, K. C., & Dennis, M. L. (2010). Characteristics, needs, services, and outcomes of youths in juvenile treatment drug courts as compared to adolescent outpatient treatment. *Drug Court Review, 7,* 10–56.

Jaffe, S. L. (1990). *Step workbook for adolescent chemical dependency recovery: A guide to the first five steps.* Washington, DC: American Psychiatric Press.

Jaffe, S. L. (2001). *Adolescent substance abuse intervention workbook: Taking a first step.* Washington, DC: American Psychiatric Press.

Jensen, C. D., Cushing, C. C., Aylward, B. S., Craig, J. T., Sorell, D. M., &, Steele, R. G. (2011). Effectiveness of motivational interviewing interventions for adolescent substance use behavior change: A meta-analytic review. *Journal of Consulting and Clinical Psychology, 79,* 433–440.

Johnston, L. D., Miech, R. A., O'Malley, P. M., Bachman, J. G., Schulenberg, J. E., & Patrick, M. E. (2018). *Monitoring the future national survey results on drug use: 1975–2017: Overview, key findings on adolescent drug use.* Ann Arbor: Institute for Social Research, University of Michigan.

Johnston, L. D., O'Malley, P. M., Bachman, J. G., & Schulenberg, J. E. (2011). *Monitoring the future: National results on adolescent drug use.* Ann Arbor: Institute for Social Research, University of Michigan.

Kaminer, Y., & Bukstein, O. G. (Eds.). (2008). *Adolescent substance abuse: Psychiatric comorbidity and high-risk behaviors*. New York: Routledge/Taylor Francis.

Kaminer, Y., Bukstein, O., & Tarter, R. E. (1991). The Teen-Addiction Severity Index: Rationale and reliability. *International Journal of the Addictions, 26,* 219–226.

Kaminer, Y., Wagner, E., Plumer, B., & Seifer, R. (1993). Validation of the teen addiction severity index (T-ASI): Preliminary findings. *American Journal on Addictions, 2,* 250–254.

Kandel, D. B., Kessler, R. C., & Margulies, R. Z. (1978). Antecedents of adolescent initiation into stages of drug use: A developmental analysis. *Journal of Youth and Adolescence, 7*(1), 13–40.

Kandel, D., & Yamaguchi, K. (2002). Stages of drug involvement in the U.S. population. In D. Kandel (Eds.), *Stages and pathways of drug involvement: Examining the gateway hypothesis* (pp. 65–89). New York: Cambridge University Press.

Katusic, S. K., Barbaresi, W. J., Colligan, R. C., Weaver, A. L., Leibson, C. L., & Jacobsen, S. J. (2005). Psychostimulant treatment and risk for substance abuse among young adults with a history of attention-deficit/hyperactivity disorder: A population-based, birth cohort study. *Journal of Child and Adolescent Psychopharmacology, 15*(5), 764–776.

Kaufman, J., Birmaher, B., Axelson, D., Pereplitchikova, F., Brent, D., & Ryan, N. (2016). *The KSADS-PL DSM-5.* Unpublished manuscript. Retrieved January 6, 2019, from *www.kennedykrieger.org/sites/default/files/library/documents/faculty/ksads-dsm-5-screener.pdf.*

Kelly, J. F., Dow, S. J., Yeterian, J. D., & Kahler, C. W. (2010). Can 12-step group participation strengthen and extend the benefits of adolescent addiction treatment?: A prospective analysis. *Drug and Alcohol Dependence, 110,* 117–125.

Kelly, J. F., Kaminer, Y., Kahler, C. W., Hoeppner, B., Yeterian, J., Cristello, J. V., & Timko, C. (2017). A pilot randomized clinical trial testing integrated 12-step facilitation (iTSF) treatment for adolescent substance use disorder. *Addiction, 109,* 766–773.

Kelly, J. F., & Myers, M. G. (2007). Adolescent's participation in Alcoholics Anonymous and Narcotics Anonymous: Review, implications and future directions. *Journal of Psychoactive Drugs, 39*(3), 259–269.

Kelly, J. F., Myers, M. G., & Brown, S. A. (2000). A multivariate process model of adolescent 12-step attendance and substance use outcome following inpatient treatment. *Psychology of Addictive Behaviors, 4,* 376–389.

Kelly, S. M., Gryczynski, J., Mitchell, S. G., Kirk, A., O'Grady, K. E., & Schwartz, R. P. (2014). Validity of brief screening instrument for adolescent tobacco, alcohol, and drug use. *Pediatrics, 133,* 819–826.

Kendall, P. C. (Ed.). (2011). *Child and adolescent therapy: Cognitive-behavioral procedures* (4th ed.). New York: Guilford Press.

Kendler, K. S., Schmitt, E., Aggen, S. H., & Prescott, C. A. (2008). Genetic and environmental influences on alcohol, caffeine, cannabis, and nicotine use from early adolescence to middle adulthood. *Archives of General Psychiatry, 65,* 674–682.

Kennard, B. D., Hughes, J. L., & Foxwell, A. A. (2016). *CBT for depression in children and adolescents: A guide to relapse prevention.* New York: Guilford Press.

Kloss, A., Weller, R. A., Chan, R., & Weller, E. B. (2009). Gender differences in adolescent substance abuse. *Current Psychiatry Reports, 11,* 120–126.

Knight, J. R., Sherritt, L., Harris, S. K., Gates, E. C., & Chang, G. (2003). Validity of brief alcohol screening tests among adolescents: A comparison of the AUDIT, POSIT, CAGE and CRAFFT. *Alcoholism, Clinical and Experimental Research, 27,* 67–73.

Knight, J. R., Sherritt, L., Shrier, L. A., Van Hook, S., Lawrence, N., Brooks, T., et al. (2002). Validity of the CRAFFT substance abuse screening test among adolescent clinic patients. *Archives of Pediatric and Adolescent Medicine, 156,* 607–614.

Kollins, S. H., McClernon, F. J., & Fuemmeler, B. F. (2005). Association between smoking and attention-deficit/hyperactivity disorder symptoms in a population-based sample of young adults. *Archives of General Psychiatry, 62,* 1142–1147.

Lee, S. S., Humphreys, K. L., Flory, K., Liu, R., & Glass, K. (2011). Prospective association of childhood attention-deficit/hyperactivity disorder (ADHD) and substance use and abuse/dependence: A meta-analytic review. *Clinical Psychology Review, 31,* 328–341.

Levy, S. J., & Kokotailo, P. K. (2011). Substance use screening, brief intervention, and referral to treatment for pediatricians. *Pediatrics, 128*(5), e1330–1340.

Levy, S. J., Siqueira, L. M., & the Committee on Substance Abuse, American Academy of Pediatrics. (2014). Testing for drugs of abuse in children and adolescents. *Pediatrics, 133,* e1798.

Levy, S. J., Williams, J. F., & the Committee on Substance Abuse and Prevention. (2016). Substance use screening, brief intervention, and referral to treatment. *Pediatrics, 138,* e20161211.

Lewis, R. A., Piercy, F. P., Sprenkle, D. H., & Trepper, T. S. (1990), Family-based interventions for helping drug-abusing adolescents. *Journal of Adolescent Research, 5,* 82–95.

Liddle, H. A. (2001). *Multidimensional family therapy for adolescent cannabis users* (Cannabis Youth Treatment Series, Vol. 5). Rockville, MD: U.S. Department of Health and Human Services, Substance Abuse and Mental Health Services Administration Center for Substance Abuse Treatment.

Liddle, H. A., & Dakof, G. A. (1995). Family-based treatment for adolescent drug use: State of the science. In E. Rahdert & D. Czechowicz (Eds.), *Adolescent drug abuse: Clinical assessment and therapeutic interventions* (NIH Publication No. 95–3908, NIDA Research Monograph Series 156) (pp. 218–254). Rockville, MD: National Institute on Drug Abuse.

Liddle, H. A., Dakof, G. A., Parker, K., Diamond, G. S., Barrett, K., & Tejeda, M. (2001). Multidimensional family therapy for adolescent substance abuse: Results of a randomized clinical trial. *American Journal of Drug and Alcohol Abuse, 27,* 651–687.

Liddle, H. A., Rowe, C. L., Dakof, G. A., Henderson, C. E., & Greenbaum, P. E. (2009). Multidimensional family therapy for young adolescent substance abuse: Twelve-month outcomes of a randomized controlled trial. *Journal of Consulting and Clinical Psychology, 77,* 12–25.

Lynskey, M. T., Agrawal, A., & Heath, A. C. (2010). Genetically informative research on adolescent substance use: Methods, findings, and challenges. *Journal of the American Academy of Child and Adolescent Psychiatry, 49,* 1202–1214.

Lynskey, M. T., & Fergusson, D. M. (1995). Childhood conduct problems, attention deficit behaviors, and adolescent alcohol, tobacco, and illicit drug use. *Journal of Abnormal Child Psychology, 23*(3), 281–302.

Mahoney, J. L., & Cairns, R. B. (1997). Do extracurricular activities protect against early school dropout? *Developmental Psychology, 33,* 241–253.

Marsch, L. A., Bickel, W. K., Badger, G. J., Stothart, M. E., Quesnel, K, J., Stanger, C., & Brooklyn, J. (2005). Comparison of pharmacological treatments for opioid-dependent adolescents: A randomized controlled trial. *Archives of General Psychiatry, 62,* 1157–1164.

Marshal, M. P., Friedman, M. S., Stall, R., King, K. M., Miles, J., Gold, M. A., et al. (2008). Sexual orientation and adolescent substance use: A meta-analysis and methodological review. *Addiction, 103,* 546–556.

Martin, C. S., Kaczynski, N. A., Maisto, S. A., Bukstein, O. M., & Moss, H. B. (1995). Patterns of DSM-IV alcohol abuse and dependence symptoms in adolescent drinkers. *Journal of Studies on Alcohol, 56,* 672–680.

Martin, C. S., Pollock, N. K., Bukstein, O. G., & Lynch, K. G. (2000). Inter-rater reliability of the SCID alcohol and substance use disorders section among adolescents. *Drug and Alcohol Dependence, 59*(2), 173–176.

Martino, S., Grilo, C. M., & Fehon, D. C. (2000). Development of the drug abuse screening test for adolescents (DAST-A). *Addictive Behaviors, 25*(1), 57–70.

Mayer J., & Filstead, W. J. (1979). The Adolescent Alcohol Involvement Scale: An instrument for measuring adolescents' use and misuse of alcohol. *Journal of Studies on Alcohol, 40,* 291–300.

McLellan, A. T., Luborsky, L., Woody, G. E., & O'Brien, C. P. (1980). An improved diagnostic evaluation instrument for substance abuse clients: The Addiction Severity Index. *Journal of Nervous and Mental Disease, 168*(1), 26–33.

Meier, M. H., Caspi, A., Ambler, A., Harrington, H. L., Houts, R., Keefe, R. S. E., et al. (2012). Persistent cannabis users show neuropsychological decline from childhood to midlife. *Proceedings of the National Academy of Sciences of the USA, 109,* E2657–2664.

Meyers, R. J., & Smith, J. E. (1995). *Clinical guide to alcohol treatment: The community reinforcement approach.* New York: Guilford Press.

Milberger, S., Biederman, J., Faraone, S., Chen, L., & Jones, J. (1997). ADHD is associated with early initiation of cigarette smoking in children and adolescents. *Journal of American Academy of Child and Adolescent Psychiatry, 36*(1), 37–44.

Miller, A. L., Rathus, J. H., & Linehan, M. (2017). *Dialectical behavior therapy with suicidal adolescents.* New York: Guilford Press.

Miller, W. R., & Rollnick, S. (2013). *Motivational interviewing: Helping people change* (3rd ed.). New York: Guilford Press.

Mitchell, S. G., Gryczynski, J., O'Grady, K. E., & Schwartz, R. P. (2013). SBIRT for adolescent drug and alcohol use: Current status and future directions. *Journal of Substance Abuse Treatment, 44*, 463–472.

Moberg, D. P., & Finch, A. J. (2008). Recovery high schools: A descriptive study of school programs and students. *Journal of Groups in Addiction and Recovery, 2*, 128–161.

Moberg, D. P., & Hahn, L. (1991). The adolescent drug involvement scale. *Journal of Adolescent Chemical Dependency, 2*(1), 75–88.

Molina, B. S., & Pelham, W. E., Jr. (2003). Childhood predictors of adolescent substance use in a longitudinal study of children with ADHD. *Journal of Abnormal Psychology, 112*, 497–507.

Moolchan, E. T., Robinson, M. L., Ernst, M., Cadet, J. L., Pickworth, W. B., Heishman, S. J., et al. (2004). Safety and efficacy of the nicotine patch and gum for the treatment of adolescent tobacco addiction. *Pediatrics, 115*, 407–414.

Naar-King, S., & Suarez, M. (2011). *Motivational interviewing with adolescents and young adults.* New York: Guilford Press.

Najavits, L. M., Gallop, R. J., & Weiss, R. D. (2006). Seeking Safety therapy for adolescent girls with PTSD and substance use disorder: A randomized controlled trial. *Journal of Behavioral Health Services and Research, 33*, 453–463.

National Institute on Alcohol Abuse and Alcoholism. (2007). *Helping patients who drink too much: A clinician's guide* (Updated 2005 edition) (NIH Publication No. 07-3769). Washington, DC: Author. Retrieved from *http://pubs.niaaa. nih.gov/publications/Practitioner/Clinicians Guide2005/guide.pdf.*

National Institute on Alcohol Abuse and Alcoholism. (2014). Alcohol Screening and Brief Intervention for Youth: A practitioner's guide. Retrieved January 3, 2015, from *http://www.niaaa.nih.gov/sites/default/files/publications/Youth-Guide.pdf.*

National Institute on Drug Abuse. (2003). *Preventing drug use among children and adolescents: A research-based guide for parents, educators, and community leaders* (2nd ed.). Rockville, MD: Author.

National Institute on Drug Abuse. (2014). Principles of adolescent substance use disorder treatment: A research-based guide. Retrieved July 7, 2014, from *www.drugabuse.gov/sites/default/files/podata_1_17_14.pdf.*

National Research Council and Institute of Medicine. (2009). *Preventing mental, emotional, and behavioral disorders among young people: Progress and possibilities.* Washington, DC: National Academies Press.

Nestler, E. J. (2005). Is there a common molecular pathway for addiction? *Nature Neurosocience, 11*, 1445–1449.

Newton, A. S., Dong, K., Mabood, N., Ata, N., Ali, S., Gokiert, R., et al. (2013). Brief emergency department interventions for youth who use alcohol and other drugs: A systematic review. *Pediatric Emergency Care, 29*, 673–684.

O'Connell, M. E., Boat, T., & Warner, K. E. (2009). *Preventing mental, emotional, and behavioral disorders among young people: Progress and possibilities.* Washington, DC: National Academies Press.

Palladino, G. (1996). *Teenagers: An American history*. New York: Basic Books.

Parker, J. G., Rubin, K. H., Price, J. M., & DeRosier, M. E. (1995). Peer relationships, child development, and adjustment: A developmental psychopathology perspective. In D. Cicchetti & D. J. Cohen (Eds.), *Wiley series on personality processes: Developmental psychopathology, Vol. 2. Risk, disorder, and adaptation* (pp. 96–161). Oxford, UK: Wiley.

Patterson, G. R., & Forgatch, M. S. (1987). *Parents and adolescents: Living together, the basics*. Eugene, OR: Castalia.

Pompili, M., Serafini, G., Innamorati, M., & Girardi, P. (2012). Substance abuse and suicide risk among adolescents. *European Archives of Psychiatry and Clinical Neuroscience, 262*, 469–485.

Prinz, R. J., & Miller, G. E. (1996). Parental engagement interventions for children at risk for conduct disorder. In R. D. Peters & R. J. McMahon (Eds.), *Preventing disorders, substance abuse, and delinquency* (pp. 161–183). Thousand Oaks, CA: SAGE.

Prochaska, J. O., & DiClemente, C. C. (1983). Stages and processes of self-change of smoking: Toward an integrative model of change. *Journal of Consulting and Clinical Psychology, 51*, 390–395.

Rathus, J. H., & Miller, A. L. (2014). *DBT® skills manual for adolescents*. New York: Guilford Press.

Robbins, M. S., Horigian, V. E., & Szapocznik, J. (2007). Brief strategic family therapy™: An empirically validated family therapy for adolescents with disruptive behavior problems. *Journal of Brief, Systemic, and Strategic Therapies, 1*(1), 39–62.

Robin, A. L., & Foster, S. L. (1989). *Negotiating parent–adolescent conflict: A behavioral-family systems approach*. New York: Guilford Press.

Rohde, P., Lewinsohn, P. M., Kahler, C. W., Seeley, J. R., & Brown, R. A. (2001). Natural course of alcohol use disorders from adolescence to young adulthood. *Journal of the American Academy of Child and Adolescent Psychiatry, 40*, 83–90.

Rowan, A. B. (2001). Adolescent substance abuse and suicide. *Depression and Anxiety, 14*, 186–191.

Rusby, J. C., Westling, E., Crowley, R., & Light, J. M. (2017). Legalization of recreational marijuana and community sales policy in Oregon: Impact on adolescent willingness and intent to use, parent use, and adolescent use. *Psychology of Addictive Behaviors, 32*, 84–92.

Ryan, S. R., Stanger, C., Thostenson, J., Whitmore, J. J., & Budney, A. J. (2013). The impact of disruptive behavior disorder on substance use treatment outcome in adolescents. *Journal of Substance Abuse Treatment, 44*, 506–514.

Sampl, S., & Kadden, R. (2001). *Motivational enhancement therapy and cognitive behavioral therapy for adolescent cannabis users: 5 sessions* (Cannabis Youth Treatment Series, Vol. 1). Rockville, MD: U.S. Department of Health and Human Services, Substance Abuse and Mental Health Services Administration Center for Substance Abuse Treatment.

Santisteban, D. A., Szapocznik, J., Perez-Vidal, A., Murray, E. J., Kurtines, W. M., & Laperriere, A. (1996). Efficacy of intervention for engaging youth and families into treatment and some variables that may contribute to differential effectiveness. *Journal of Family Psychology, 10,* 35–44.

Santisteban, D. A., Tejeda, M., Dominicis, C., & Szapocznik, J. (1999). An efficient tool for screening for maladaptive family functioning in adolescent drug abusers: The Problem Oriented Screening Instrument for Teenagers. *American Journal of Drug and Alcohol Abuse, 25*(2), 197–206.

Slesnick, N., & Prestopnik, J. L. (2004). Office- versus home-based family therapy for runaway, alcohol-abusing adolescents: Examination of factors associated with treatment attendance. *Alcoholism Treatment Quarterly, 22,* 3–19.

Smith, D. C., & Hall, J. A. (2007). Strengths-oriented referral for teens (SORT): Giving balanced feedback to teens and families. *Health and Social Work, 32,* 69–72.

Smith, D. C., Hall, J. A., Williams, J. K., An, H., & Gotman, N. (2006). Comparative efficacy of family and group treatment for adolescent substance abuse. *American Journal on Addictions, 15,* 131–136.

Smith, G. T., Goldman, M. S., Greenbaum, P. E., & Christiansen, B. A. (1995). Expectancy for social facilitation from drinking: The divergent paths of high-expectancy and low-expectancy adolescents. *Journal of Abnormal Psychology, 104,* 32–40.

Smith, T. E., Sells, S. P., Rodman, J., & Reynolds, L. R. (2006). Reducing adolescent substance abuse and delinquency: Pilot research of a family oriented psycho-education curriculum. *Journal of Child and Adolescent Substance Abuse, 15,* 105–115.

Spear, L. P. (2002). The adolescent brain and the college drinker: Biological basis of propensity to use and misuse alcohol. *Journal of Studies on Alcohol, 14*(Suppl.), 71–81.

Spirito, A., Esposito-Smythers, C., Wolff, J., & Uhl, K. (2011). Cognitive-behavioral therapy for adolescent depression and suicidality. *Child and Adolescent Psychiatric Clinics of North America, 20*(2), 191–204.

Stanger, C., & Budney, A. J. (2010). Contingency management approaches for adolescent substance use disorders. *Child and Adolescent Psychiatric Clinics of North America, 19,* 47–62.

Stanger, C., Ryan, S. R., Fu, H., Landes, R. D., Jones, B. A., Bickel, W. K., et al. (2012). Delay discounting predicts adolescent substance abuse treatment outcome. *Experimental and Clinical Psychopharmacology, 20*(3), 205–212.

Steinberg, L. (2005). Cognitive and affective development in adolescence: Cognitive and affective development in adolescence. *Trends in Cognitive Sciences, 9*(2), 69–74.

Steinberg, L., Dahl, R. E., Keating, D., Kupfer, D. J., Masten, A. S., & Pine, D. S. (2006). Psychopathology in adolescence: Integrating affective neuroscience with the study of context. In D. Cicchetti & D. J. Cohen (Eds.), *Developmental psychopathology: Vol. 2. Developmental neuroscience* (2nd ed., pp. 710–741). New York: Wiley.

Steinberg, L., Elmen, J. D., & Mounts, N. S. (1989). Authoritative parenting, psychosocial maturity, and academic success among adolescents. *Child Development, 60,* 1424–1436.

Steinberg, L., Fletcher, A., & Darling, N. (1994). Parental monitoring and peer influences on adolescent substance use. *Pediatrics, 93,* 1060–1064.

Stevens, S. J., Schwebel, R., & Ruiz, B. (2007). The seven challenges: An effective treatment for adolescents with co-occurring substance abuse and mental health problems. *Journal of Social Work Practice in the Addictions, 7*(3), 29–49.

Stinchfield, R. D. (1997). Reliability of adolescent self-reported pretreatment alcohol and other drug use. *Substance Use and Misuse, 32,* 63–76.

Stinchfield, R. D. (2010). A critical review of adolescent problem gambling assessment instruments. *International Journal of Adolescent Medicine and Health, 22,* 77–93.

Substance Abuse and Mental Health Services Administration. (2001). *Adolescent cannabis users, motivational enhancement and cognitive behavioral therapy* (Cannabis Youth Treatment Series, Vol. 1). Rockville, MD: Author.

Substance Abuse and Mental Health Services Administration. (2008). *Results from the 2007 National Household Survey on Drug Use and Health: National findings.* Rockville, MD: Author.

Substance Abuse and Mental Health Services Administration. (2013). *Results from the 2012 National Survey on Drug Use and Health: Summary of national findings* (NSDUH Series H-46, HHS Publication No. [SMA] 13-4795). Rockville, MD: Author.

Substance Abuse and Mental Health Services Administration. (2017). *Key substance use and mental health indicators in the United States: Results from the 2016 National Survey on Drug Use and Health* (NSDUH Series H-52, HHS Publication No. [SMA] 17-5044). Rockville, MD: Author. Retrieved August 29, 2018, from *www.samhsa.gov/data.*

Sung, M., Erkanli, A., Angold, A., & Costello, E. J. (2004). Effects of age at first substance use and psychiatric comorbidity on the development of substance use disorders. *Drug and Alcohol Dependence, 75,* 287–299.

Swendsen, J., Burstein, M., Case, B., Conway, K. P., Dierker, L., He, J., & Merikangas, K. R. (2012). Use and abuse of alcohol and illicit drugs in U.S. adolescents. *Archives of General Psychiatry, 69,* 390–398.

Szapocznik, J., Kurtines, W. M., Foote, F., Perez-Vidal, A., & Hervis, O. (1986). Conjoint versus one-person family therapy: Further evidence for the effectiveness of conducting family therapy through one person with drug-abusing adolescents. *Journal of Consulting and Clinical Psychology, 54,* 395–397.

Szapocznik, J., Perez-Vidal, A., Briskman, A. L., Foote, F. H., Santisteban, D., & Hervis, O. (1988). Engaging adolescent drug abusers and their families in treatment. *Journal of Consulting Clinical Psychology, 56,* 552–557.

Szapocznik, J., & Williams, R. A. (2000). Brief strategic family therapy: Twenty-five years of interplay among theory, research and practice in adolescent behavior problems and drug abuse. *Clinical Child and Family Psychology Review, 3,* 117–134.

Szobot, C. M., Rohde, L. A., Katz, B., Ruaro, P., Schaefer, T., Walcher, M., et al. (2008). A randomized crossover clinical study showing that methylphenidate-SODAS improves attention-deficit/hyperactivity disorder symptoms in adolescents with substance use disorder. *Brazilian Journal of Medical and Biological Research, 41,* 250–257.

Tait, R. J., & Hulse, G. K. (2003). A systematic review of the effectiveness of brief interventions with substance using adolescents by type of drug. *Drug and Alcohol Review, 22*, 337–346.

Tanner-Smith, E. E., Wilson, S. J., & Lipsey, M. W. (2013). The comparative effectiveness of outpatient treatment for adolescent substance abuse: A meta-analysis. *Journal of Substance Abuse Treatment, 44*, 145–158.

Tapert, S. F., & Brown, S. A. (1999). Neuropsychological correlates of adolescent substance abuse: Four-year outcomes. *Journal of the International Neuropsychological Society, 5*, 481–493.

Tapert, S. F., & Brown, S. A. (2000). Substance dependence, family history of alcohol dependence, and neuropsychological functioning in adolescence. *Addictions, 95*(7), 1043–1053.

Tarter, R. E. (1990). Evaluation and treatment of adolescent substance abuse: A decision tree method. *American Journal of Drug Alcohol Abuse, 16*(1&2), 1–46.

Thurstone, C., Riggs, P. D., Salomonsen-Sautel, S., & Mikulich-Gilbertson, S. K. (2010). Randomized, controlled trial of atomoxetine for attention-deficit/hyperactivity disorder in adolescents with substance use disorder. *Journal of the American Academy of Child and Adolescent Psychiatry, 49*, 573–582.

Tomlinson, K. L., Brown, S. A., & Abrantes, A. (2004). Psychiatric comorbidity and substance use treatment outcomes of adolescents. *Psychology of Addictive Behaviors, 18*(2), 160–169.

Upadhyaya, H. P., Brady, K. T., & Wang, W. (2004). Bupropion SR in adolescents with comorbid ADHD and nicotine dependence: A pilot study. *Journal of the American Academy of Child and Adolescent Psychiatry, 43*, 199–205.

Upadhyaya, H. P., Deas, D., & Brady, K. T. (2005). A practical clinical approach to the treatment of nicotine dependence in adolescents. *Journal of the American Academy of Child and Adolescent Psychiatry, 44*, 942–946.

U.S. Department of Health and Human Services, Substance Abuse and Mental Health Administration. (2009). Risk and protective factors for mental, emotional, and behavioral disorders across the life cycle. Retrieved from *http://dhss.alaska.gov/dbh/Documents/Prevention/programs/spfsig/pdfs/IOM_Matrix_8%205x11_FINAL.pdf.*

Waldron, H. B., & Kaminer, Y. (2004). On the learning curve: The emerging evidence supporting cognitive-behavioral therapies for adolescent substance abuse. *Addiction, 99*(Suppl. 2), 93–105.

Waldron, H. B., Slesnick, N., Turner, C. W., Brody, J. L., & Peterson, T. (2001). Treatment outcomes for adolescent substance abuse at 4- and 7-month assessments. *Journal of Consulting and Clinical Psychology, 69*, 802–813.

Waldron, H. B., & Turner, C. W. (2008). Evidence-based psychosocial treatments for adolescent substance abuse. *Journal of Clinical Child and Adolescent Psychology, 37*, 238–261.

Walton, M. A., Chermack, S. T., Shope, J. T., Bingham, C. R., Zimmerman, M. A., Blow, F. C., & Cunningham, R. M. (2010). Effects of a brief intervention for reducing violence and alcohol misuse among adolescents: A randomized controlled trial. *Journal of the American Medical Association, 304*, 527–535.

Webb, C., Scudder, M., Kaminer, Y., & Kadden, R. (2001). *The motivational enhancement therapy and cognitive behavioral therapy supplement: 7 sessions of cognitive behavioral therapy for adolescent cannabis users* (Cannabis Youth Treatment Series, Vol. 2). Rockville, MD: U.S. Department of Health and Human Services, Substance Abuse and Mental Health Services Administration Center for Substance Abuse Treatment.

White, A. M., Jordan, J. D., Schroeder, K. M., Acheson, S. K., Georgi, B. D., Sauls, G., et al. (2004). Predictors of relapse during treatment and treatment completion among marijuana-dependent adolescents in an intensive outpatient substance abuse program. *Substance Abuse, 25*, 53–59.

White, H. R., & Labouvie, E. W. (1989). Towards the assessment of adolescent problem drinking. *Journal of Studies on Alcohol, 50*, 30–37.

Wilens, T. E. (2007). The nature of the relationship between attention-deficit/ hyperactivity disorder and substance use. *Journal of Clinical Psychiatry, 68*(1), 4–8.

Wilens, T. E., Vitulano, M., Upadhyaya, H., Adamson, J., Sawtelle, R., Utzinger, L., et al. (2008). Cigarette smoking associated with attention deficit hyperactivity disorder. *Journal of Pediatrics, 15*, 414–419.

Williams, R. J., & Chang, S. Y. (2000). Addiction Centre Adolescent Research Group: A comprehensive and comparative review of adolescent substance abuse treatment outcome. *Clinical Psychology Science and Practice, 7*, 138–166.

Windle, M., Spear, L. P., Fuligni, A. J., Angold, A., Brown, J. D., Pine, D., et al. (2008). Transitions into underage and problem drinking: Developmental processes and mechanisms between 10 and 15 years of age. *Pediatrics, 121*, 273–289.

Winters, K. C. (1992). Development of an adolescent alcohol and other drug abuse screening scale: Personal Experience Screening Questionnaire. *Addictive Behaviors, 17*, 479–490.

Winters, K. C., Botzet, A. M., Fahnhorst, T., & Koskey, R. (2009). Adolescent substance abuse treatment: A review of evidence-based research. In C. Leukefeld, T. Gullotta, & M. Staton Tindall (Eds.), *Handbook on the prevention and treatment of substance abuse in adolescence* (pp. 73–96). New York: Springer Academic.

Winters, K. C., Fahnhorst, T., Botzet, A., Lee, S., & Lalone, B. (2012). Brief intervention for drug-abusing adolescents in a school setting: Outcomes and mediating factors. *Journal of Substance Abuse Treatment, 42*, 279–288.

Winters, K. C., & Henly, G. (1993). *Adolescent diagnostic interview and manual.* Los Angeles: Western Psychological Services.

Winters, K. C., & Kaminer, Y. (2008). Screening and assessing adolescent substance use disorders in clinical populations. *Journal of the American Academy of Child and Adolescent Psychiatry, 47*, 740–744.

Winters, K. C., Martin, C. S., & Chung, T. (2011). Substance use disorders in DSM-V when applied to adolescents. *Addiction, 106*, 882–887.

Winters, K. C., Stinchfield, R. D., Henly, G. A., & Schwartz, R. H. (1991). Validity of adolescent self-report of alcohol and other drug involvement. *International Journal of Addictions, 25*, 1379–1395.

Winters, K., Stinchfield, R. D., Henly, G. A., & Schwartz, R. H. (1996). Convergent and predictive validity of the Personal Experience Inventory. *Journal of Child and Adolescent Substance Abuse, 5,* 37–55.

Winters, K. C., Stinchfield, R. D., & Opland, E. (2000). The effectiveness of the Minnesota Model approach in the treatment of adolescent drug abusers. *Addiction, 65,* 601–612.

Woody, G., Poole, S. A., Subramaniam, G. A., Dugosh, K., Bogenschutz, M., Abbott, P., et al. (2008). Extended vs. short-term buprenorphine/naloxone for treatment of opioid-addicted youth: A randomized trial. *Journal of the American Medical Association, 300,* 2003–2011.

Index

Note. *f* or *t* following a page number indicates a figure or a table.

ABC model, 124–129, 125*f*, 133, 134
Abstinence, 94, 95–96, 147–149
Abuse, 119, 164
Academic performance, 5, 45, 94, 95–96, 178. *See also* School functioning
Acceptance, 27, 112–113
Addiction Severity Index, 78–79
Adolescent Alcohol Involvement Scale (AAIS), 74
Adolescent community reinforcement approach (A-CRA), 10*t*, 109
Adolescent Drinking Index (ADI), 74
Adventure therapy, 108
Advice, 39–40, 101, 102
Affirmations. *See also* OARS acronym
  change and, 33, 35, 38
  motivational interviewing (MI) and, 25, 40
  resistance and, 27
Aftercare interventions, 13, 108–109. *See also* Treatment
Alcohol use, 2, 4, 66–67, 67*f*, 226
Alcohol Use Disorders Identification Test (AUDIT), 74
Alcoholics Anonymous (AA), 13, 109, 112–115
Alternative peer-group (APG) programs, 110–111
Ambivalence, 23–24, 38–39, 40, 41
Anger management, 218, 220*t*, 222–223

Antecedents in the ABC model, 124–129, 125*f*, 132–134, 135*f*–136*f*, 169. *See also* Triggers for use and relapse
Anxiety, 121–122, 222*t*, 224, 228–229
Arguing, 27, 38
Assessment. *See also* Screening
  comorbidity and, 212
  comprehensive assessment, 78–91, 79*t*, 83*t*
  confidentiality and, 53–54
  domain model of, 78–89, 79*t*, 83*t*
  drug testing, 62–63, 64*t*
  effective treatments and, 96
  instruments for, 89–91
  interviewing and engaging adolescents, 56–62, 58*t*, 61*t*
  overview, 44–45, 64, 91
  parental involvement in, 54–56
  referrals for or initiating, 45–53
Attention-deficit/hyperactivity disorder (ADHD), 210, 227–228
Automatic thoughts, 145. *See also* Thoughts

Behavioral management, 217–224, 220*t*, 221*t*, 222*t*
Behavioral patterns
  ABC model and, 124–129, 125*f*, 132–134, 135*f*–136*f*
  assessment and, 79*t*, 80–81
  brief interventions (BIs) and, 101

cognitive-behavioral therapy (CBT) and, 121–123
effective treatments and, 95–96
emotional factors and, 209–210
levels of care and, 99
screening and assessment and, 58
Beliefs, 20, 40–41
Booster sessions, 105
Brainstorming, 30, 31, 139, 140–141
Brief interventions (BIs). *See also* Treatment
feedback on the results of screenings and, 76–77
motivational interviewing (MI) and, 39–40
overview, 9, 11, 101–115
Brief Screener for Tobacco, Alcohol and other Drugs (BSTAD), 68
Brief screening, 66–74, 67*f*, 69*f*. *See also* Screening
Brief strategic family therapy (BSFT), 10*t*, 12, 164–165

Cannabis Youth Treatment (CYT) study, 12
Change
brief interventions (BIs) and, 101
comorbidity and, 213
confidence in the ability for, 121
levels of care and, 99
motivational interviewing (MI) and, 23–24
planning for, 36–39, 36*t*
readiness for, 30–31, 31*f*, 35–36, 35*t*, 40, 61*t*
stages of, 61*t*
Change plan, 36–39, 36*t*, 103–104, 105
Change talk, 24, 31–32, 32, 34*t*, 104–105
Choice, 27, 38, 40
Chores, 178
Clinical interviews, 56–62, 58*t*, 61*t*. *See also* Assessment
Clinicians
brief interventions (BIs) and, 101
cognitive-behavioral therapy (CBT) and, 123, 130–131
cultural factors and, 117–120
empathy and, 18–19
group treatment and, 116–117
integrated practices and, 211
motivational interviewing (MI) and, 24
overview, 92–93
parent and family motivation and engagement, 18–20

parent management training (PMT) · and, 170, 171
parent–adolescent problem solving (PAPS) training and, 193–194
referrals for screening and assessment from parents and, 51–53
Coercion, 21–23, 97
Cognitive factors, 20, 99, 121–122, 123, 126. *See also* Thoughts
Cognitive-behavioral therapy (CBT). *See also* Treatment
behavioral and emotional management and, 217–224, 220*t*, 221*t*, 222*t*
clinician skills and roles, 130–131
comorbidity and, 211, 217–224, 220*t*, 221*t*, 222*t*
components of, 122–129, 125*f*, 129*f*
coping and refusal skills and, 142–149
crisis control, 149–152
identifying triggers, 132–134, 135*f*–136*f*
integrated treatment practices and, 214
overview, 10*t*, 12, 121–122, 130, 163
problem solving and, 134, 137–142, 142*f*
session topics and structure, 131–132, 131*t*
skills building and, 152–160, 158*f*
troubleshooting, 160–163
Collaborative approaches, 23, 43, 212
Communication, 94, 184–185, 184*t*, 207. *See also* Communication skills training; Negotiation
Communication skills training. *See also* Communication; Negotiation
family interventions and, 165
parent management training (PMT) and, 166, 169, 178, 182–186, 183*t*, 184*t*
parent–adolescent problem solving (PAPS) training and, 189–191, 194
Community-based treatment, 13, 100
Community-level risk and protective factors, 4–5, 7*t*. *See also* Risk factors
Comorbidity. *See also* Dual treatment; Psychiatric disorders; Psychopathology
assessment and, 87–88
cognitive-behavioral therapy (CBT) and, 162
effective treatments and, 94, 96
integrated practices and, 210–229, 220*t*, 221*t*, 222*t*

Comorbidity *(cont.)*
  overview, 209–210, 230
  pharmacological treatments and,
    226–229
  psychoeducation and, 225–226
  referrals for screening and assessment
    from, 48–49
  treatment and, 120, 212–215
Compliance, lack of, 27, 41, 177–178, 202.
    See also Resistance
Concurrent treatment, 213. *See also*
    Comorbidity; Integrated SUD
    treatment; Treatment
Confidence change talk, 32, 33, 34*t*, 121.
    See also Change talk
Confidence ruler, 30, 31*f*
Confidentiality, 53–54, 64, 77–78
Consequences
  ABC model and, 124–129, 125*f*, 132–134,
    135*f*–136*f*, 169
  assessment and, 82, 84–85
  contingency management and, 41–43
  parent management training (PMT)
    and, 169, 178–179, 179*t*
  problem solving and, 140
  of substance use, 39–40
Contingencies, 122
Contingency contracts, 187. *See also*
    Contracts
Contingency management (CM). *See also*
    Treatment
  developing contracts and, 186–188
  drug testing and, 62–63
  overview, 12, 41–43
  parent management training (PMT)
    and, 169, 180–182, 181*t*
Continuum of care, 211–212. *See also* Levels
    of care; Treatment
Contracts, 169, 186–188, 189–190, 201,
    204–205
Control, 27, 86–87
Coordination of care, 211
Coping skills, 142–149
CRAFFT screening tool, 50, 68–74, 69*f*,
    72*f*
Cravings, 87, 144–145, 149, 229
Criminal justice system, 45. *See also*
    Juvenile justice system; Legal factors
Crisis control, 149–152
Criticism, 153–154
Cultural factors, 117–120

Danger, 53–54, 96, 99. *See also* Safety
DARN acronym, 32
Decision making, 4, 40, 110–111
Decisional balance, 29–30, 29*f*
Delinquency, 5, 65–66. *See also* Juvenile
    justice system
Denial, 17–18, 27, 51–53
Depression
  cognitive-behavioral therapy (CBT) and,
    121–122
  integrated treatment practices and,
    213–214, 221*t*, 223–224
  overview, 210
  risk and protective factors and, 4
Developmental factors
  assessment and, 79–80
  parent management training (PMT)
    and, 169, 170–172, 171*t*
  risk and protective factors and, 4, 5
Diagnosis, 2–4, 3, 211–212
*Diagnostic and Statistical Manual of Mental
    Disorders* (DSM-III-R, DSM-IV, DSM-
    IV-TR, DSM-5), 3, 81, 86, 90
Dialectical behavioral therapy (DBT), 144,
    224
Disciplinary practices, 5, 164, 169, 176–
    180, 179*t*. *See also* Punishments
Disease model, 112–113, 163
Distraction techniques, 144, 146–147
Distress tolerance, 224
Domain model of assessment, 78–89, 79*t*,
    83*t*, 96. *See also* Assessment
Drug courts, 22, 41
Drug testing, 62–63, 64*t*, 91. *See also*
    Assessment; Screening
Drug Use Screening Inventory (DUSI),
    74, 90
Dual treatment, 210. *See also* Comorbidity;
    Integrated SUD treatment; Treatment
Duration of treatment, 111–112

EARS acronym, 33
Elaboration techniques, 30, 33, 35
Emergency department (ED), 50, 73
Emotions
  behavioral problems and, 209–210
  cognitive-behavioral therapy (CBT) and,
    121–123
  emotional management, 217–224, 220*t*,
    221*t*, 222*t*
  functional analysis of, 132–134, 135*f*–136*f*

levels of care and, 99
triggers for use and relapse, 125–126,
125*t*
Empathy
brief interventions (BIs) and, 102
comorbidity and, 215
motivational interviewing (MI) and,
39–40
OARS acronym and, 24–27
parent and family motivation and
engagement, 18–19, 40
planning for change and, 37–38
Employment functioning, 79*t*, 84, 89,
95–96
Engagement
comorbidity and, 212
cultural factors and, 117–120
effective treatments and, 94
motivational interviewing (MI) and, 40
parent and family motivation and
engagement, 18–23, 40, 55–56
screening and assessment and, 56–62,
58*t*, 61*t*
Environmental factors
alternative peer-group (APG) programs
and, 110–111
levels of care and, 99
risk and protective factors and, 4–5
screening and assessment and, 58
triggers for use and relapse, 126
Ethnicity, 117–118
Evidence-based treatments and practices.
See also Treatment
duration of treatment and, 111–112
effective treatments, 93–96, 95*t*
overview, 7–13, 10*t*, 15–16, 231–232
Evocative approaches, 23, 31–36, 34*t*, 35*t*
Expert trap, 38–39
Externalizing symptoms, 214, 218–219

Family factors, 5, 6*t*, 19–20, 79*t*, 85, 88,
95–96. *See also* Risk factors
Family involvement in treatment, 18–23,
40–41, 94, 113–114
Family support network, 10*t*
Family therapies. *See also* Parent
management training (PMT); Parent-
adolescent problem solving (PAPS)
training; Treatment
elements of, 165–168
family systems therapy, 164–165

modifications to PAPS training and,
207–208
overview, 10*t*, 11–12, 164–165, 188, 208
Feedback, 39–40, 101–102, 104–105, 122
Feelings, 121–123, 132–134, 135*f*–136*f*. *See
also* Emotions
Financial factors, 111–112, 115
Fishbowl technique, 42–43
Flexibility, 104–105
FRAMES acronym, 39–40, 101–103. *See
also* Brief interventions (BIs)
Functional analysis, 122–123, 124–129,
125*f*, 132–134, 135*f*–136*f*
Functional family therapy (FFT), 10*t*,
11–12, 164–165

GAIN assessment instrument, 90
Gender, 1, 119, 119–120
Goals. *See also* Treatment planning
effective treatments and, 94
motivational interviewing (MI) with
families and parents and, 40, 41
parent management training (PMT)
and, 169, 170–172, 171*t*
planning for change and, 36–39, 36*t*
Group treatment, 113, 115–117, 124. *See
also* Treatment
Guiding process, 28–31, 29*f*, 31*f*

Happiness scale, 155–156
Harm reduction approaches, 94
Health care settings, 49–50, 66
Health habits, 4, 213
Home-based interventions, 99
Homework (school), 178
Homework (treatment)
cognitive-behavioral therapy (CBT) and,
122, 134, 138
coping and refusal skills and, 149
parent management training (PMT)
and, 172, 173, 175, 180, 182, 186
Household responsibilities, 178. *See also*
Responsibility

Impulsivity, 134, 137
Incentives, 42–43, 180–182, 181*t*
Integrated SUD treatment. *See also* Dual
treatment; Treatment
behavioral and emotional management
and, 217–224, 220*t*, 221*t*, 222*t*
identifying triggers, 224

Integrated SUD treatment *(cont.)*
  integrated behavioral and family
    therapy model, 164–165
  levels of care and, 99
  motivation and, 215–217
  overview, 210–229, 220*t*, 221*t*, 222*t*, 230,
    231–232
  pharmacological treatments and,
    226–229
  prosocial activities and peers, 225
  psychoeducation and, 225–226
Intensive outpatient (IOP) treatment
    model, 10*t*, 107, 109
Internalizing symptoms, 214, 217–218
Interpersonal factors, 95–96, 125–126,
    125*t*, 152–153. *See also* Peer
    relationships; Social factors
Interventions. *See also* Motivational
    interviewing (MI); Treatment;
    Treatment planning
  aftercare interventions, 13
  brief interventions (BIs), 9, 11
  contingency management and, 41–43
  evidence-based treatments and
    practices, 7–9
  feedback on the results of screenings
    and, 76–77
Interviews, 56–62, 58*t*, 61*t*. *See also*
    Assessment
Intoxication, 99
Involuntary commitment, 22–23

Juvenile justice system, 22, 45, 48–49.
    See also Criminal justice system;
    Delinquency; Legal factors

Labeling trap, 38–39
Lapses, 150–151, 162–163. *See also* Relapse
    prevention
Learning, 123, 130
Legal factors, 3, 22–23, 62–63, 65–66. *See
    also* Criminal justice system; Juvenile
    justice system
Levels of care, 98–100, 211–212. *See also*
    Treatment
LGBT adolescents, 119–120
Listening, reflective. *See* Reflective
    listening

Managed care, 111–112
Medical care settings, 49–50, 66
Medical factors, 79*t*, 89, 99

Medication. *See* Pharmacological treatments
Mental health treatment, 46–47, 99. *See
    also* Treatment
Menu (treatment options), 39–40, 102
Mindfulness, 144, 224
Modeling
  cognitive-behavioral therapy (CBT) and,
    122, 133–134, 141–142
  coping and refusal skills and, 148–149
  parent management training (PMT)
    and, 185–186
Monitoring
  effective treatments and, 94
  parent management training (PMT)
    and, 169, 172–175, 178
  risk and protective factors and, 5
Mood disorders, 210, 228–229. *See also*
    Depression
Motivation. *See also* Motivational
    interviewing (MI)
  brief interventions (BIs) and, 101,
    104–105
  cognitive-behavioral therapy (CBT) and,
    123
  comorbidity and, 213
  contingency management and, 41–43
  cultural factors and, 117–120
  effective treatments and, 94
  integrated treatment practices and,
    215–217
  overview, 17–18, 43, 121
  parent and family motivation and
    engagement, 18–23
  parent management training (PMT)
    and, 166–168
Motivational enhancement therapy (MET),
    10*t*, 112–113, 122
Motivational interviewing (MI). *See also*
    OARS acronym
  brief interventions (BIs) and, 39–40,
    101, 104–105
  comorbidity and, 215–217
  engaging process and, 24–28
  evoking process and, 31–36, 34*t*, 35*t*
  with families and parents, 40–41
  guiding process and, 28–31, 29*f*, 31*f*
  overview, 10*t*, 23–41, 29*f*, 31*f*, 34*t*, 35*t*, 36*t*
  parent management training (PMT)
    and, 168, 170–171
  planning and, 36–39, 36*t*
  screening and assessment and, 61, 73
Motivation-based interventions, 106

Multidimensional family therapy (MDFT), 10*t*, 12, 164–165
Multidimensional treatment foster care (MTFC), 10*t*
Multifamily groups, 113–114
Multisystemic therapy (MST), 10*t*, 12, 96, 164–165

Narcotics Anonymous (NA), 13, 109, 112–115
Negative consequences. *See also* Consequences
  assessment and, 82, 84–85
  cognitive-behavioral therapy (CBT) and, 146
  functional analysis of, 132–134, 135*f*–136*f*
  harm reduction approaches and, 94
  parent management training (PMT) and, 169, 176–180, 179*t*
  problem solving and, 140
Negative reinforcement, 41–43, 62–63. *See also* Reinforcement
Negotiation. *See also* Communication; Communication skills training; Parent–adolescent problem solving (PAPS) training
  alcohol and drug use and, 202–204
  change plan and, 37–38
  guidelines for, 194*t*–195*t*
  at home, 204–205
  initial training session, 194–196, 195*f*, 196*t*, 197–198, 199–201
  modifications to PAPS training and, 207–208
  overview, 189, 190–191

OARS acronym. *See also* Affirmations; Motivational interviewing (MI); Open-ended questions; Reflective listening; Summaries
  brief interventions (BIs) and, 104–105
  comorbidity and, 215–217
  evoking process and, 31
  guiding process and, 28
  overview, 24–27
  parent management training (PMT) and, 168
Open-ended questions, 24, 61. *See also* OARS acronym
Outcomes, 7–9, 117–120
Outpatient treatment, 106–107, 115. *See also* Treatment

Palmer Drug Abuse Program (PDAP), 110–111
Parent management training (PMT). *See also* Family therapies
  communication skills and, 182–186, 183*t*, 184*t*
  developing contracts and, 186–188
  discipline and negative consequences and, 176–180, 179*t*
  goal setting and, 170–172, 171*t*
  introducing to clients, 170–172, 171*t*
  monitoring and tracking, 172–175
  overview, 165–168, 188
  parent–adolescent problem solving (PAPS) training and, 198
  session topics and structure, 169, 169*t*
  use of positive reinforcement, rewards, and contingency management, 180–182, 181*t*
Parent–adolescent problem solving (PAPS) training. *See also* Family therapies
  alcohol and drug use and, 202–204
  after the initial training session, 202
  initial training session, 194–201, 195*f*, 196*t*
  modification of, 207–208
  negotiation and, 189, 190–191, 194*t*–195*t*, 204–205
  overview, 189–191, 208
  role of the clinician and, 193–194
  session topics and structure, 191, 193
  troubleshooting, 205–207
Parental involvement, 18–23, 40–41, 105, 113–114, 131
Parent–child relationship, 4, 164
Parenting with Love and Limits (PLL), 10*t*
Parents
  parenting skills, 5, 171–172, 171*t*
  referrals for screening and assessment from, 50–53
  resistance and, 205–206
  screening and assessment and, 54–56, 64
  with SUDs, 164
  supervision and. See Supervision
  treatment and, 97–98
Patterns of use
  cognitive-behavioral therapy (CBT) and, 121–122
  frequency of use, 71
  functional analysis of, 124–129, 125*f*
  overview, 2–4
  parent–adolescent problem solving (PAPS) training and, 202–204

Patterns of use *(cont.)*
  relapse prevention and management,
    149–152
  risk and protective factors and, 5
  screening and assessment and, 58*t*,
    59–62, 61*t*, 79*t*, 82, 84, 86–87
  triggers for use and relapse, 125–126,
    125*t*
Peer relationships. *See also* Social factors
  alternative peer-group (APG) programs
    and, 110–111
  assessment and, 79*t*, 85, 88–89
  cognitive-behavioral therapy (CBT) and,
    154–160, 158*f*
  cultural factors and, 118
  risk and protective factors and, 5, 6*t*,
    59, 60
  treatment and, 94, 95–96, 225
Pharmacological treatments, 13–15, 94,
    226–229. *See also* Treatment
Placement decisions, 98–100
Planning, 36–39, 36*t*, 150–151. *See also*
    Treatment planning
Planning to use, 86–87
Pleasant activities, 156–157, 158*f*
Positive consequences, 132–134,
    135*f*–136*f*, 140, 154–156, 169. *See also*
    Consequences
Positive reinforcement, 41–43, 62–63,
    73–74, 180–182, 181*t*. *See also*
    Reinforcement
Prevention, 232, 233*t*–234*t*
Primary care system, 49–50, 66
Problem Oriented Screening Instrument
    for Teenagers (POSIT), 74, 90
Problem solving
  cognitive-behavioral therapy (CBT) and,
    134, 137– 142, 142*f*
  effective treatments and, 94
  family interventions and, 165
  integrated treatment practices and,
    218–219
  introducing to clients, 138–141
  motivational interviewing (MI) with
    families and parents and, 40
  negotiations at home and, 204–205
  parent management training (PMT)
    and, 169, 187–188
  parent–adolescent problem solving
    (PAPS) training and, 194–201, 195*f*,
    196*t*, 204–205
  twelve-step approaches and, 113

Prosocial activities, 79*t*, 110–111, 223–224,
    225
Prosocial behaviors, 94, 95, 154–160, 158*f*,
    213
Protective factors, 4–7, 6*t*–7*t*
Psychiatric disorders. *See also* Comorbidity;
    Psychopathology
  assessment and, 79*t*, 87–88
  effective treatments and, 94, 95–96
  evidence-based treatments and
    practices, 8–9
  gender and treatment and, 119
  integrated treatment practices and,
    212–229, 220*t*, 221*t*, 222*t*
  levels of care and, 99
  pharmacological treatments and, 13–15,
    226–229
  risk and protective factors and, 4
Psychoeducation, 12, 164, 225–226
Psychopathology. *See* Comorbidity;
    Psychiatric disorders
Psychosocial functioning, 8, 94–95
Punishments, 41–43, 62–63, 177. *See also*
    Disciplinary practices

Race, 117–118
Rapport, 40, 101
Readiness for change. *See* Change
Recovery skills, 86–87, 105, 188, 190–191
Recreational activities, 79*t*, 156–157, 158*f*
Referrals, 45–53, 64, 93
Reflection, 27, 33, 35, 40
Reflective listening, 25–26, 38, 40, 61. *See
    also* OARS acronym
Reframing techniques, 27, 30, 40
Refusal skills, 113, 142–149
Reinforcement
  cognitive-behavioral therapy (CBT) and,
    147
  contingency management and, 41–43
  drug testing and, 62–63
  parent management training (PMT)
    and, 180–182, 181*t*
  prosocial behavior and, 154–156
  reinforcer sampling, 156–157
  reinforcers, 181, 181*t*
  screening and, 73–74
Relapse potential, 99, 125–126, 125*t*, 162–163
Relapse prevention
  cognitive-behavioral therapy (CBT) and,
    149–152, 162–163
  comorbidity and, 213

effective treatments and, 94
integrated treatment practices and, 224
twelve-step approaches and, 113
Residential treatment, 21–22, 99, 100, 107–108, 115
Resistance
cognitive-behavioral therapy (CBT) and, 160–161
motivational interviewing (MI) and, 27–28, 38–39, 40
parent and family motivation and engagement, 20, 40
parent–adolescent problem solving (PAPS) training and, 205–206
planning for change and, 38
Responsibility, 39–40, 102, 112–113, 178
Rewards, 41–43, 62–63, 180–182, 181*t*
Risk factors. *See also* Triggers for use and relapse
overview, 4–7, 6*t*–7*t*, 232, 235
screening and assessment and, 46, 60
treatment and, 8, 96, 120, 228
Role plays
cognitive-behavioral therapy (CBT) and, 130, 133–134, 141–142
coping and refusal skills and, 148–149
parent management training (PMT) and, 175, 179, 180, 182, 185–186
parent–adolescent problem solving (PAPS) training and, 196
Rules, 167–168, 176–180, 179*t*
Rutgers Alcohol Problem Index (RAPI), 74

Safety, 53–54, 96, 98, 99, 227–228
Scaling confidence, 30, 31*f*
Schedule for Affective Disorders and Schizophrenia for School-Age Children (K-SADS), 90
School functioning. *See also* Academic performance
assessment and, 79*t*, 84, 88–89
effective treatments and, 94, 95–96
evidence-based treatments and practices, 8
parent management training (PMT) and, 178
School referrals, 47–48. *See also* Referrals
School-based interventions, 99
Screening. *See also* Assessment
brief screening, 66–74, 67*f*, 69*f*
confidentiality and, 53–54
CRAFFT screening tool, 50, 68–74, 69*f*, 72*f*

drug testing, 62–63, 64*t*
feedback on the results of, 75–78
interviewing and engaging adolescents, 56–62, 58*t*, 61*t*
overview, 44–45, 64, 65–78, 67*f*, 69*f*, 72*f*, 91
parental involvement in, 54–56
referrals for or initiating, 45–53
standardized screening instruments, 74, 79*t*
Screening, brief intervention, and referral to treatment (SBIRT) programs, 11, 66–67, 76–77, 101
Screening to Brief Intervention (S2BI) tool, 68, 71–73, 72*f*
Seeking Safety, 10*t*, 224
Self-efficacy
brief interventions (BIs) and, 102–103
motivational interviewing (MI) and, 30–31, 31*f*, 39–40
parent and family motivation and engagement, 20
parent management training (PMT) and, 166–168
planning for change and, 38
Self-help groups, 94, 144
Self-medication, 119, 210
Self-report, 56–62, 58*t*, 61*t*
Sequential model of treatment, 96. *See also* Treatment
Seven Challenges® Program, 10*t*
Sexual behavior, 80
Sexual orientation, 119–120
Skills-based interventions
cognitive-behavioral therapy (CBT) and, 141–149, 152–160, 158*f*
coping and refusal skills and, 142–149
group treatment and, 117
overview, 4, 122–123, 129, 129*f*
parent management training (PMT) and, 166–168
twelve-step approaches and, 113
Social factors. *See also* Peer relationships
alternative peer-group (APG) programs and, 110–111
assessment and, 79*t*
levels of care and, 99
pharmacological treatments and, 226
risk and protective factors and, 5
social skills, 94, 113
support from others and, 30, 144, 147, 157, 159, 226

Social factors *(cont.)*
  triggers for use and relapse, 125–126, 125*t*
Social learning model, 168
Stages of change. *See* Change
Student assistance programs (SAPs), 47–48
Substance use disorders (SUDs) in general
  overview, 231–232, 235
  prevalence of adolescent substance use and misuse and, 3–4
  resources regarding, 237–239
  risk and protective factors and, 4–7, 6*t*–7*t*
Substance use patterns. *See* Patterns of use
Suicidal behavior, 213, 224
Summaries, 26–27, 33, 35. *See also* OARS acronym
Supervision, 94, 169, 228
Sustain talk, 24

Targets of change, 122, 197–199. *See also* Goals
Teen Addiction Severity Index (T-ASI), 74, 90
Teen Intervene, 10*t*
Therapeutic communities (TCs), 108
Thoughts, 121–123, 132–134, 135*f*–136*f*, 145–147. *See also* Cognitive factors
Time-line follow-back (TLFB) method, 82, 90–91
Token economy, 182. *See also* Contingency management (CM); Reinforcement
Tolerance, 87
Tracking of behavior, 169, 172–175
Training of clinicians, 130–131. *See also* Clinicians
Trauma, 119, 210, 224
Treatment. *See also* Brief interventions (BIs); Cognitive-behavioral therapy (CBT); Dual treatment; Family therapies; Interventions; Pharmacological treatments; Treatment planning; Twelve-step approaches
  coercion and, 21–23
  comorbidity and, 210–229, 220*t*, 221*t*, 222*t*
  effective treatments, 93–96, 95*t*

evidence-based treatments and practices, 7–9
  group treatment, 115–117
  history of, 87
  levels of care, 98–100
  motivation and, 18
  overview, 9–13, 10*t*
  referrals for screening and assessment and, 46–47
  resources for, 237–239
  responding to parent concerns regarding, 97–98
Treatment planning. *See also* Treatment
  cultural factors and, 117–120
  effective treatments, 95*t*
  integrated practices and, 212–215
  levels of care, 98–100
  overview, 92, 120
  responding to parent concerns regarding, 97–98
Triggers for use and relapse. *See also* Antecedents in the ABC model; Risk factors
  coping and refusal skills and, 144–149
  crisis control, 149–152
  functional analysis of, 135*f*–136*f*, 124–129, 125*f*, 132–134
  identification of, 224
  integrated treatment practices and, 224
  overview, 125–126, 125*t*
  problem solving and, 137, 139–141
  skills building and, 129, 129*f*
Twelve-step approaches, 13, 109, 112–115

Urges, 144–145
Urine screening, 62, 63, 64*t*, 91. *See also* Drug testing
Use patterns. *See* Patterns of use

Values, 41, 86
Vocational functioning, 79*t*, 84, 89, 95–96

Wilderness therapy, 108
Withdrawal symptoms, 86, 99, 229
Work functioning, 79*t*, 84, 89, 95–96